UNSTILL

Praise For

Unstill

Lenny Gallo's book, *Unstill,* dives deep into how torturous akathisia and medication-induced movement disorders can be for an individual. With Lenny's artistic abilities and descriptiveness, he will indeed pull the reader into real-life scenarios while he takes you on his journey of persistence. Highly recommended—this is an important memoir to anyone currently questioning their mental health.

— Akathisia Alliance

Though the issues presented are those of gravitas, Lenny Gallo's incredible writing style offers a pathway through the crippling clutch of almost any disorder for which there are no answers. He speaks to the life of many millions for whom chronic anxiety has become a limiting, dream-crushing way of life—all the while entertainingly guiding us down a path of adaptive living. Mr. Gallo further reveals clear medical failures and deficiencies while navigating the pharmaceutical cornucopia that is today's North America. This memoir is destined to become an inspiration for sufferers and adventurers alike. It is a testament to human resiliency and the possibilities that truly lie within anyone's reach.

— Cary Harrison
KPFK Los Angeles Public Radio Host

Reading a memoir is to peer into the unknown of someone's life and see that person in a completely different light. Writing a memoir is to pull back the curtain with the hope you can change or touch a reader with your own experiences. Therapist and author Lenny Gallo has done just that in an entertaining, witty, and honest account that uses humor and art to shed light on mental health. *Unstill* is both a creative outlet and an exquisite extension of storytelling. I highly recommend this book for anyone who has ever questioned their own mental health, considered taking medication, and who needs to see they are not alone.

— Gregory G. Allen
award-winning writer, filmmaker, advocate

In recent years, mental health has risen to a higher position in our cultural awareness. However, maneuvering through the system is too often confusing and can result in feelings of disconnection and alienation. In his memoir author, Lenny Gallo, gives us a powerful, honest, and vulnerable account of his experiences and the unfortunate consequences he endured.

—Patrick Hughes, LCSW

A beautiful, heartfelt memoir that can only be told by the person who lived it. Life doesn't always give us what we expect; there are many twists and turns that shape us into the people we eventually become. Lenny's memoir serves as a warning for anyone considering medications to deal with their mental health and shows the persistence of the human spirit. Well worth the read.

—Lee D. Britton
Author of *Faith and Hope and Tragedy*

UNSTILL

The Ordeal of Anxiety, Pills,
and an Undiagnosed Disorder

A Memoir

by Lenny Gallo

L. R. Fin Media & Publications
New Jersey

L. R. Fin Media & Publications
P.O. Box 84
Verona, NJ 07044

ISBN 979-8-9904725-0-1 (hardcover)
ISBN 979-8-9904725-4-9 (paperback)
ISBN 979-8-9904725-1-8 (special edition color paperback)
ISBN 979-8-9904725-2-5 (eBook)
ISBN 979-8-9904725-3-2 (audio)

LCCN: 2024909669

Publisher's Cataloging-in-Publication data

Names: Gallo, Lenny, author.
Title: Unstill : the ordeal of anxiety , pills , and an undiagnosed disorder : a memoir / by Lenny Gallo.
Description: Verona, NJ: L.R. Fin Media & Publishing, 2024.
Identifiers: LCCN: 2024909669 | ISBN: 979-8-9904725-0-1 (hardcover) | 979-8-9904725-4-9 (paperback) | 979-8-9904725-1-8 (special edition color paperback) | 979-8-9904725-2-5 (eBook) | 979-8-9904725-3-2 (audio)
Subjects: LCSH Gallo, Lenny. | Mentally ill--United States--Biography. | Anxiety--Patients--United States--Biography. | Artists--Biography. | Movement disorders--Patients--Biography. | BISAC BIOGRAPHY & AUTOBIOGRAPHY / Memoirs | BIOGRAPHY & AUTOBIOGRAPHY / Medical | BIOGRAPHY & AUTOBIOGRAPHY / Artists, Architects, Photographers
Classification: LCC RC464.G35 2024 | DDC 362.2/092--dc23

First Hardcover Edition: October 1, 2024

Book Editors: Sondra Beaulieu, Louise D. Stahl, and Don Weise
Cover Art & Paintings: Lenny Gallo
Cover & Book Design: Glen Edelstein, Hudson Valley Book Design
www.LennyGallo.com

To all those who still struggle with no answers.

Contents

Author's Note

What do you do when, suddenly, your life gets thrown upside down and an entity enters that takes over and uproots everything you know? I never thought I'd have to figure that out. Shortly over a decade ago, I developed a bizarre movement disorder that forced me to re-examine every aspect of myself. This condition, set in motion by the side effects of medication, presented itself as mental health issues combined with physical components.

Writing this book has been an almost four-year journey I never intended to take. I thought it would be a piece of me that I would carry in secret, with only a few select friends and family aware of the full details. It felt too personal, shameful, and embarrassing. But, when confronted for the second time with some of the demons described in this book, I began to think that it was worth sharing this experience with the world. My partner, Scott, and my friend Nick, both of whom you will read about in this book, encouraged me. They realized, even more than I had begun to, that it was important information for others to know.

My journey with this piece began with the art in this book, created during the time of the ordeal. I am a conceptual artist at heart. Over the years, those who have seen artwork from this period in my life often asked me to explain it. They said, "It's too abstract," or, "I don't get it." I think it's a fair request to ask an artist to explain their artwork and the rationale behind it. As I started to write artist's mini statements to caption each work, memories that had been repressed for a long time began to surface. These remembrances and the artist's statements took on a life of their own, and stories shaped and blended one into another. Unfortunately, for legal reasons, some of the art and titles in this book have been censored to adhere to copyright and trademark laws. During the time of this nightmare, that was the last thing on my mind.

Through this process, I was forced to reflect on what led to my bizarre disorder. Memories arose of what it was like to grow up with my mother, who herself had mental health problems. There were the memories of growing up gay. My strongest reactions, though, were those that happened right before and during the course of the worst times of the movement disorder: the medications I put into my body, and the doctors who didn't know what was going on—or who just wouldn't listen.

As a talk therapist, I am an avid believer in exposure therapy: having people confront their fears. The best way for me to continue my mental health journey, I concluded, would be to tell my story, reflect on it, and hopefully begin the process of changing the narrative. I didn't want to live with these thoughts in my head anymore or hold onto those memories. They will always be a part of me, but I wanted to move beyond them and the power they had over me.

So why should you read this tale?

I felt so alone when my condition began. Perhaps you are struggling with some of the symptoms listed in this book. If you are, I will caution you that some of the material may trigger you. Maybe you struggle with anxiety, or perhaps you're taking mental health medication or are thinking about taking it. It's possible that you have encountered the side effects of medications. A lot of people are experiencing the disorders I describe, and I hope that if you are one of them, my story will make you feel less alone—less crazy.

This is by no means a how-to book. For legal reasons, I must tell you that this book does not provide any medical advice and should not be taken as medical advice or a substitute for medical doctors' instructions. This is my journey, and this is how I have come to understand and navigate it. This may not be everyone's journey. You should work with trusted professionals if you are struggling with the conditions listed in this book, or with anything that requires medical attention. I do offer some thoughts and opinions on this disorder and some resources at the end for those who want to research further. Additionally, all the names of doctors, friends, and others mentioned in this book are changed, and the identities of individuals have been altered to protect their identity. Some names of places have been changed as well.

But what if you don't have a movement disorder or mental health issues? Why should you read this book? It is a cautionary tale, and I believe that at some point in everyone's life we are forced to confront a demon so powerful and robust that it will require one to reflect on every aspect of oneself and rip you from your core. It enters when you least expect it and saps your energy. The demon will be different for all, but you'll know it's there because it cannot be ignored. My hope is that this book will lead you to question your relationship with doctors and medication and that you will be encouraged by some common experience in my story of resilience and perseverance.

PART I

"Anyone who goes to a psychiatrist should have his head examined."
—Samuel Goldwyn, film producer

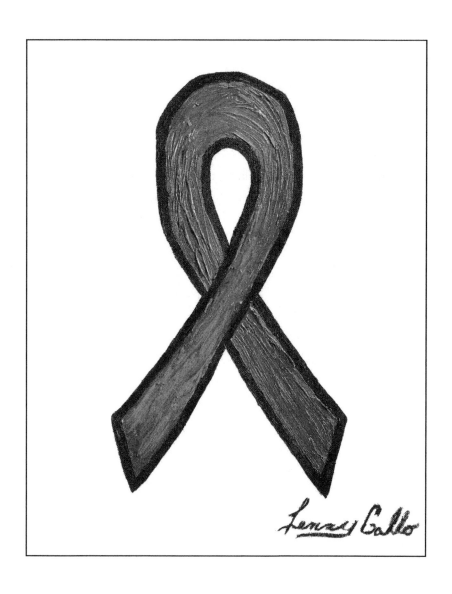

Mental Health Awareness, 2012, oil on canvas, 14" x 18".

Prologue

I've been trying all day not to look but by noon the anxiety is too much. I pull down my pants, and, as I've done for the past few weeks now, assume the position and squat on the bathroom floor. The handheld mirror in my left hand is positioned at just the right angle to get a clearer view of my anus. I think to myself, *Oh, God, it's still there. Why is it still here?*

My dermatologist told me last week that I have a fungal infection, which may be yeast. I didn't even know men could get yeast infections.

How the fuck did I get a yeast infection in my ass?

"Seriously?" I say to God, as I look up at the bathroom ceiling. "Now this?!"

Part of my anxiety stems from everything I have read on the Internet that indicates this might be chronic. My big fear of the day: *What if I have to go on heavy-duty meds to treat this thing? How will they interact with the other meds I'm on?*

Medicine and I have a very mixed relationship.

"Honey, can you look at my ass?" I yell at Scott, my life partner, who is doing work in his office adjacent to the bathroom.

"What?" he shouts back.

He comes into the bathroom and tries not to laugh when he sees the contorted pose I have gotten myself into.

"Don't laugh, just look at it," I say.

"What am I looking for?" he asks.

"Has the redness gone down?"

I'm now doggy style, cheeks spread as far as I can pull them, hoping he will notice something that I haven't.

Trying to hold back his laughter, Scott answers. "It looks fine."

Of course, no fucking help! Why do I even ask you?

"It's still there. I can see it when I look at it in this light," I say. I want him to go down the rabbit hole of my anxiety with me, not minimize it. But Scott isn't fazed by these sorts of things. It's not who he is. A grapefruit could be growing out of the side of his neck, and he wouldn't worry an ounce. He knows not to fuel my anxiety and is always able to remain calm when I want to catastrophize the situation.

"You're going to be fine!" he shouts as he leaves the bathroom, shaking his head.

When he's gone, I begin breathing exercises, inhaling deeply, and exhaling, trying to release the tension that is throughout my body. I remind myself of things that I've learned: time will give me answers and let me know what the status of my rear end will be. I know that right now I can't get the information I would like. And the fact of the matter is that there is nothing I can do. I must wait and see what happens with the creams my dermatologist prescribed for me.

Always fucking waiting and seeing. I can never just get clear, straight answers.

No, don't go there, I remind myself. *You've gotten through way worse before; you can do this.*

After a pseudo examination of myself, which really consists of me just looking more intently at the redness and trying to will it away, I go outside, have a cigarette, and continue to try and calm myself. My mind wants to go to the place where my thoughts loop in my brain.

I've been in that place before and I try to fight it. But today it's sending me into a fit of anxiety.

As I stand outside smoking, I think: *You're going to be fine. You're going to get through this. It's just yeast. You've got yeast. You love yeast in its bread form. Just breathe. Be still.* But my efforts at trying to calm myself down are failing. *Who the fuck am I kidding? Today is not going to be a still kind of day.*

This seems like the appropriate place to mention that my editors, friends, and family wanted me to cut this yeast infection anecdote, citing that it's too divisive, crass, bizarre. Normally I would agree, but it isn't a prurient story about yeast in my ass. When I was younger, I would have seen it for what it was: something that would need time to clear up. No, this ordeal with the yeast infection is *really* about how it might affect another condition.

My *other* condition. Ugh. I must sound like some gay drama queen who's a hypochondriac. Many of my friends still see me that way. That's fair: for some of my life I probably was that person.

I wonder if anyone else can ever fully comprehend how something as insignificant as a yeast infection could create such turmoil in the mind. But when I get sick or have a rash or anything in my body that needs attention, my present-day forty-one-year-old self is compelled to weigh it out to determine how it might affect my other demon, and how it could impact the rest of my life.

My *other* condition begins to act up. I notice my body ticking. It often acts up when I get too lost in my head or too overwhelmed.

I'll bet you would like to know what this other condition is. So would I. It's been with me for so long, I think I understand parts of it. I recognize on an intellectual level that it's a neurological condition that causes uncontrolled movements. But there are emotional and psychological components to this thing, and there are parts of it that perhaps I will never know.

When it acts up, I often think back to when it first started. I'm reminded of the time I had to spend a weekend in a psych ward, trying

5

to figure out if I was sane. And there was the hopelessness I felt for days when the movements first invaded my body. I had to deal with doctors who didn't know what was going on with me. There were the pills, and endless hours of moving, pacing, and ticking; always wondering when and if it would stop and go away. It was such an uncertain time.

This fucking condition. It has a name; it actually has several. But the minute I name it, nobody knows what I'm talking about, and that doesn't do justice to it. It's like a beast or demon that has attached itself to me; but that sounds too cliché, even though that is what it often feels like. I call it Edmund, similar to the character Edmund in Shakespeare's tragedy *King Lear*. My Edmund is the equivalent of an illegitimate brother brought into my life, who attempts to take over to gain power. In Shakespeare's play, Edmund orders the death of protagonists and plots to murder his father and brother, but he tells the audience in his soliloquy how misunderstood he is. *Entitled shit.* I do feel bad for the poor guy, however. Shakespeare doesn't give us much about his childhood, but it would appear that he didn't always have it easy. I can certainly relate to that.

Perhaps if you understand my Edmund, you'll see why the pesky parasite in my ass has me on edge.

But in order to understand Edmund, you must first understand what allowed him to exist and what life was like before. A fungal infection may have triggered Edmund today, but he had been gestating in my soul for years; probably when the robin first laid her eggs.

I didn't always move uncontrollably. At one time my life had stillness in it, although I wasn't always aware or appreciative of it. The Edmund that is attached at my hip today is a product of a lifetime of buried and suppressed anxiety that was mishandled and misguided.

I hate the word *anxiety*. It has kept me in therapy most of my adult life, and it's a good friend of Edmund. I know that everyone has anxiety; I am no exception. For me, anxiety is a feeling of impending doom, yet it often has no basis in reality. Anxiety is the body's way of signaling you to take action. To combat this wretched feeling, people often turn to the act of worrying in an effort to pretend that they are doing something about their anxiety. We know that worrying serves no purpose other than to give the illusion of control over situations that are often far outside the realm of one's jurisdiction. The reason some people get bouts of uncontrollable anxiety and others do not can depend on a lot of factors: situational, environmental, genetic. I can certainly pinpoint parts of my anxiety to my mother.

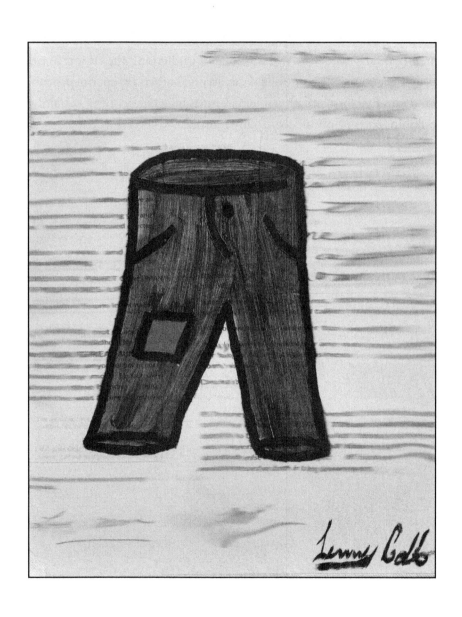

Mom's Bad Genes, 2012, mixed media, 11" x 14".

CHAPTER 1

Mom's Bad Genes

Mom and my early childhood probably laid the foundation for Edmund. Back then, Mom was a heavyset Italian woman who struggled with anxiety and a panic disorder her entire life. While the diagnoses doctors gave her were anxiety and panic disorder, I often suspected that there was more behind her mental health that I never understood. She had long, dark brown hair, smelled of Chanel No. 5, and wore those standard '80s glasses that covered way too much of her face. She always wore bright red or pink lipstick, which, even then, I could tell was not the best choice for her and made her look almost clown-like. But it was the eighties and nineties. She often told me that she grew up in an abusive and unreliable household, was locked in closets, and physically and verbally abused, which I'm sure traumatized her. From what I could tell from research I did years later, mental health issues seemed to be genetic on her side of the family. As a kid, I remember asking about grandpa, who had passed away before I was born. My mother told me that "he went away to the crazy house," but not much more was revealed to me about his condition.

Mom was always taking different medications for her mental health, but none of them ever appeared to work. Her fears of impending doom dominated my childhood, and she did not exhibit the qualities one would associate with a loving mother. She didn't want kids. That was made very clear when I was five or six years old. I was sitting in the passenger seat riding with her one day in our grey family van, and she began to tell me the story of how I was almost not to be.

"I was going to have an abortion," she said quite casually, as if it were nothing more than a cavity that had to get filled. "I went to the clinic," she continued, "but the day I went, all these protestors were outside, so I decided not to do it. Your father was the one who wanted you guys."

I was confused and didn't know what to think or how to respond, but something felt strangely awkward inside. My uneasy thoughts were fixated on the fact that she didn't want me.

Then why did you have me? I thought, unsure of what to do with this unknown feeling inside me.

When my dad got home from work that day, I shared what Mom had told me. He covered his face with both hands and then said, "She told you that?" Dad rubbed my back and tried to find the words to explain this secret that he thought would go to the grave with him. Shaking his head in disbelief, he told me, "Don't listen to her. We wanted you … I wanted you."

With Mom, you never knew what you were getting, and even worse, what kind of mood she would be in. Her anxiety, as the doctors called it, often came out as anger. It had the typical worry and panic, but there was an angry component that left me on edge most days. Everything could be going well. I would be playing some made-up game with my younger brother. Suddenly, out of nowhere, Mom would explode into a rage because of some trivial thing, like a piece of laundry that didn't make its way into the hamper or a toy that hadn't been "properly" put away.

"Why can't either of you ever listen to me?" she would wail, tears falling from her eyes. My brother and I would freeze and look at each other, scared of what might come next, each of us secretly hoping that it wasn't our piece of clothing or toy.

This wasn't a typical clean-up-your-mess kind of mom response that other kids would experience; this was a visceral rage that seemed to emanate from her very core. "You're both an embarrassment, and you should be ashamed," she screamed as she stared into our eyes with a stern intensity that would scare Satan himself. My brother and I hung our heads down and exhibited the shame demanded of us. What else could we do? That piece of laundry that hadn't been put in the hamper or the toy that hadn't been put away represented an entire lifetime of hurt that she was unable to resolve. The only way she knew how to deal with it was to try and control the ones she could.

I rarely remember Mom attending family functions with us. She had no problem expressing her opinions to me: "I hate your dad's side of the family," she often told me with bitterness. As for vacations: "I can't travel that far—my anxiety," she shouted at my father. "Why do you always ask when you know I can't go?" My dad often hung his head down in shame, too. He just wanted some sense of normalcy for his children and himself.

As a kid, it was always hard to understand why Mom could never do any of the things that other moms seemed to do so effortlessly, like picking my brother and me up from school. Some days she would come, some days she wouldn't.

When her mother, who lived with us in her later years, passed away, a deep sadness overtook Mom that added to her emotional instability. Some days I saw her crying at the kitchen table for what seemed like an endless amount of time.

I often feared my mother, but a natural human instinct kicked in, and it pained me to see another person hurting. Going over to her, I would put my hand on hers, and softly say, "Mom, don't cry. It will be all right."

She would turn to me, listlessly, with a bitter, almost empty stare and not respond. My mother was lost in her head.

Work for her was definitely out of the question, but she liked to spend lots of money—money that we didn't have. She would want to fix the house or buy things to give her temporary moments of happiness. To support my mom's spending habits, my dad worked constantly.

Dad was a tall man, and everyone loved him the moment they met him. He had one of the most genuine smiles you ever saw and a laid-back personality. How the two of them got together is beyond me. He could make friends with just about anyone he encountered. I can't think of a single person who disliked my father. He started off as a musician. I remember as a child going to a few of his wedding and Saint Patrick's Day gigs, watching him play his heart out at the piano. During family functions, he would bust out his accordion and entertain everyone with cheesy polka tunes—such a big ham! But he was also a humble and frugal man who always seemed to love life.

My dad always picked up the slack where Mom left off in the parenting department and gave my brother and me the best childhood he could. When the life of a musician wasn't cutting it with the bills, and as my mother's never-ending quest for more things continued, he decided to become a nurse. I remember going to his nursing school graduation. He tried to teach me to use this very fancy camera to get a few pictures of him walking down the aisle. "Just push this button when you see me walking down the aisle," he told me as we stood in the auditorium filled with spectators.

My eyes lit up when I held that camera. Dad always entrusted me with big-people tasks and never steered away from giving me such responsibilities. After all, who else was going to do it? Certainly not his wife. Excited to play with this fancy toy, I must have taken one thousand pictures. I think I got some blurry shots of him getting his diploma, but none worth keeping as memorabilia.

As Dad ventured into a more traditional work world, my brother and I were left in Mom's care most of the time. You could tell Mom and Dad were never happy. Mom was always very jealous of him because he seemed to be able to easily do so many things she couldn't. My brother and I often sat on the stairs, peering down to the first floor, trying to get a glimpse of what was going on. The only time I ever saw my dad angry was when he was around my mother. "What about me?" she screamed at him. "What the fuck do you want me to do?" Dad shouted back. My brother and I looked at each other scared, confused, unsure of what to do, trying to decipher what we were seeing. I was never able to put into context these random bits of screaming.

When you grow up in a household with constant fighting and arguing, you learn to start solving problems on your own with a naïve, childlike mindset.

Unfortunately, I ended up inheriting some of Mom's bad genes, and I was primed for the events that would follow later in my life.

While I'm sure I showed signs of anxiety prior to this, the first time I remember using worry as a way of coping was about age seven. My parents had a bungalow-style house on the Northside of Chicago. Most of my days were spent playing with the neighborhood kids or hanging out at their homes. I had a few close friends, girls, who always seemed easier to connect with than boys. Playing with dolls and make-believe was way more appealing than sports. I would constantly be out of the house trying to avoid my mother.

Often, I hung out with one of my close girlfriends and spent most of my days with her. I don't know how we managed to connect, but she had a strong demeanor, and I latched on. I think I clung to her partially because of her confidence. It almost felt protective. She had a strength that seemed so foreign to me.

One day, I came home from playing with her and noticed that a robin had created a nest and laid her eggs in a nook adjacent to the entrance of our front doorway. I climbed up on a ledge and saw that the eggs had already hatched, and the babies were chirping.

How had I not seen this? I thought, jumping up to get a closer view.

In my excitement, I ran inside to tell my mother about the seemingly unique opportunity to have a close-up view of these new living beings. She came outside with me, and I pointed to the nest. Her fists clenched, and her eyes widened. That was all I needed to see to realize that she was unhappy with these birds making a home so close to the entrance of our house. Her mood and state of mind changed from calm to anger and fear. "They'll fly in, get rid of them," she repeated over and over, going back inside the house, sucking the excitement out of the moment.

"Why?" I asked her. "Let them stay."

"Get rid of them, I don't want them flying in!" What little patience she had grew thinner with my insistence that they should remain. My mother asked me several more times to move the nest to a place that was far away from the entrance of the house, but a primal part of me told me not to touch it, and I ignored her. My mother never liked it when I didn't listen to her, and her anger intensified.

"Mom, they won't fly in. I promise," I told her as if I could control the birds and get them to do my bidding. After several failed attempts of me trying to get her to see my perspective, in her most forceful and stern tone she screamed, "*Get-them-down-now!*" Then she gave me *the look*.

Most of the time, I was genuinely terrified of my mother and her unpredictability. When she gave me *the look*, I knew there was no more negotiation. If I didn't listen to her, this would not end well for me. She had no problem grabbing me by the arm and smacking me with all her force. I had felt that all too often before. Her long, fake, press-on nails would dig into my ass. Like Pavlov's dog, all I needed was a cue to listen. I caved in, got up on the ledge, lifted the tightly packed nest with the baby birds, which were no more than a few days old, and moved it to a different space, away from the entrance.

I was seven years old and knew very little about birds. The mother flew away when I approached the nest, and I wanted to make sure she could find it. I put the nest in a well-lit, sunny space just inside a flowerbed at the front of our house, thinking she would have no trouble finding it there. But that was the moment worry started to settle in. These birds now felt like my responsibility to care for.

The birds chirped away, calling out to their mother. They seemed to be asking, "Mom, where are you?" I couldn't sleep and I kept worrying and thinking about these birds. *Did I put them in a space where she could find them? She must have found them by now. Are they hungry? Maybe I should feed them.* I wanted to go out and check on the babies, but I wasn't allowed outside at this time of night, and I didn't dare wake my mother for this.

When I got worried as a child, I would turn to my mind to self-soothe. Bedtime was my favorite part of the day because I could let my imagination run wild and create fantasies that would take me away. I could get lost in my head for hours. All that night I envisioned that *The Smurfs* took me into their village and brought me on as one of their own, taking me away from the worries and uncertainty of my current reality. As I fantasized about what my life would be like as a Smurf, I finally managed to fall asleep.

The following day when I woke up, the chirping had stopped, but I heard another sound. It was from a full-grown robin, sitting just outside my window, cawing at what seemed to be me. Her look gave me a feeling in the pit of my stomach, one that I only felt when I had done something wrong: guilt. I ran downstairs and outside to check on the baby birds, only to find a squirrel rummaging around an empty nest. The robin continued to squawk at me as if to say, "Murderer! You murdered my children, you bastard!"

I asked my dad what had happened, and he said that the baby birds must have flown away. I knew he was lying and told me this just to make me feel better. The squirrel had gotten its dinner that night.

"*What did I do?*" I chastised myself, believing I had just committed the worst sin possible. Thoughts raced through my head; energy pulsed through my body; my heart was beating faster. I didn't have a word for it at the time, but I have come to understand it as anxiety. From that point on, that awful energy of anxiety penetrated my body, and worry became part of my daily existence. I was anxious and worried about everything.

I worried about school: *What the hell am I going to do for a science experiment for this stupid class project?*

I worried about some of the evil teachers at the Catholic school I attended. I would watch in terror as one of my grade school teachers slammed a student's desk across the room or grabbed a student by the shirt collar and took them into the hallway to be yelled at when they weren't obeying. I wondered: *Why is she so mean?*

I worried about if I was gay . . . Actually, I never worried about being gay; I always knew. From the moment I came out of the womb, it was clear that I liked dick. There was a day when I was walking home from school through the alleys of Chicago, and I noticed that someone had stupidly thrown out a box of old '70s porn magazines. I picked one up and stood there in the alley admiring the male physique of this muscular leather daddy with his classic porno mustache. Intrigued, my eyes were fixated on him. He stared back at me in a way that made me feel very good.

But what would happen if people found out? Would I get teased more than I already had? Beaten up? What to do?

Already I had trouble connecting with the boys in school. They were all so rough and aggressive and they liked girls. I tried to like girls in the same way they did, and I even tried engaging with the boys by doing the things they liked: soccer, softball, and basketball.

Once, during a soccer game, I was standing mid-court. The ball had been passed to me, and I actually caught it in-between my legs. My body stood there frozen. Never before had the ball come my way, and here it was, right between my legs. The spectators and other players were screaming with excitement, "Kick it in the net! Kick it in the net!"

I looked behind me; I looked in front of me. The smell of gross, young, sweaty boys filled the auditorium. All I heard was "Kick it in the net!" Going forward seemed to be the easiest way to the net. I ran and kicked that ball with my tiny legs, made it all the way to the net, and I kicked that sucker right in. What a relief when I saw that ball get in! I jumped with excitement at what would probably be a once-in-a-lifetime accomplishment. But my attention soon shifted to the disappointed shouts of the spectators.

"That fucking kid," someone said.

I stood there confused. The other team was celebrating my victorious kick. My coach walked over to me, grabbed me by the shoulder, and gave me a stern look. "You just got it in *their* team's net . . . you want the *other* net," he told me as he pointed to the correct side of the court.

Oops.

That evening, the team went out to eat pizza. None of the other boys talked to me as I sat there alone with my thoughts and the debilitating energy of anxiety.

Most boys were so different from me. I started to fear every boy I encountered, and the part of me that liked other boys in a different type of way only made that fear worse. There was really nobody I could talk to about this, so I kept it to myself.

But in these moments, my mind would keep wandering back to that day when I stood in the alley with that porno magazine. I wished I had the courage to take it. I wanted that image in front of me again: it was time to move on from *The Smurfs*.

In middle school, students were tasked with going through newspapers to collect articles on HIV to learn more about the epidemic that was overtaking the world. We just had to collect them and turn them in. After we handed in our articles, my teacher at the time proceeded to give us a lecture on the topic of being gay and HIV.

"It's okay if you're gay," she told the class in a tranquil tone. Her eyes scanned the class as she continued, "But it's only okay if you don't *act* on it. And look at these articles you've been collecting. If you're gay, you'll end up getting HIV." The teacher's eyes locked with mine, and she stared directly at me, fixated on me. Smiling insincerely, she asked, "You don't want to get HIV, do you?" My chest tightened, and my face reflected terror. I wondered if she knew my secret, and now I had something else to worry about. Sitting at my desk, I felt as though I couldn't move. I waited for her eyes to stop looking at me. All I could do was clench my fists together in an attempt to calm myself down. I desperately wanted to get out of that room.

Am I going to get HIV because I'm gay? Am I going to die? I asked myself, feeling the vibration of my racing heartbeat. *Does she know I'm gay? What if she tells my parents? My mother?*

The list of things to worry about continued to grow. Unlike Mom's anxiety, mine was never as paralyzing or angry, but each time I found something to worry about, I could feel the sense of panic build up inside of me. With anxiety, there is always something to worry about. It's like your brain won't let you find moments of peace. You have a ton of thoughts invading your head or you get fixated on asking yourself existential questions that have no answers. It becomes quite daunting.

To my dad's credit, he did everything in his power to make sure that I would not end up like my mother. He sensed my anxiety and always encouraged me to fight through my distress. At the age of fourteen, right before I was about to go off to high school, he sat me down and told me I would be taking the bus to school.

"You gotta do it," he said, looking at me, seeing that I was not happy.

"Why?" I asked, frustrated that he couldn't just drive me like he did everywhere else.

"Because I don't want you ending up like your mother."

My anxiety would have been unmanageable in my early adolescence had it not been for the support of my dad. I could always go to him, run my thoughts by him, and he never made me feel bad. But even more than the support of my dad, what really helped me manage my anxiety was finding art and theatre.

As a kid, my exposure to theatre and art was minimal and mostly superficial. My dad insisted that I play the trumpet, and in grade school I had fun as part of the school's production of *A Christmas Carol*; all of us who wanted to be in the show were cast in one role or another. In a pottery class, my friend and I got kicked out when we stole pottery that was better than what we had made. Even after he entered the nursing profession, my dad continued to play piano every day. I became familiar with his favorite ragtime and jazz standards. The only musicals I saw were the classic ones, like *The Sound of Music* and *The Wizard of Oz*, which came on TV every year. I had no idea that art galleries existed. Fortunately for me, fate intervened later, and I developed a deeper and more meaningful connection to the arts.

My dad helped me fill out the application for Lane Tech, a public school in Chicago. I didn't really have a choice on where I was going to high school. The girls I hung out with in grade school were all going to the local Catholic all-girls high school. Dad couldn't afford to send me to a private school, so Lane Tech was my only option.

My worry and anxiety were constantly on the lookout for signs of danger, and sirens went off in my head when it came to Lane. In grade school, where I was in a class of twenty-five students, I had my few girlfriends. Yes, I was getting picked on somewhat, but I had learned how to avoid conflict and keep it mostly at bay. Now, I would be attending the largest high school in Chicago, which housed several thousand teenagers, and I wouldn't know anyone.

When my anxious mind heard Chicago Public School, I thought of gang violence, drugs, getting beaten up. How was little gay me going to survive that?

"What do you want to major in?" my dad asked as he sat hunched over a desk in our family room, filling out the application for my new high school. He was checking off boxes and stopped to look up at me, waiting for my response. I started to walk away, yelling, "Major, what kind of high school requires a major?"

"This one," Dad said, tapping his foot impatiently as he waited for my response. I started to leave the room.

"Get back here, we have to do this," he said.

I stopped and huffed at him. "I don't know." My eyes rolled, and then shot daggers at him. I didn't want to deal with this. Dad's insistence on an answer made my heart race. As I often did when I was anxious,

I tried to avoid and not think about the situation that triggered it. The thought of high school had been pushed out of my mind, but standing there in front of my dad made this moment feel all too real.

"You have to pick one," he told me.

Okay, Lenny, think. Major, major . . . This feels very important. What do I want to do for the rest of my life? I didn't think I would have to deal with this until at least my second year of college. Ugh . . . why is he making me think about this? Wait, what are the choices?

"What are my choices?" I asked him.

"Drafting?" Dad said, reading from the sheet of options.

"What's that?"

He shook his head indicating that he didn't know. If neither one of us knew what it was, then the answer was clear.

"Nope."

Frustrated, he rubbed his forehead and took a deep breath. "How about math."

Just stab me in the eye. Who the hell picks math?

My chest was tightening up. "No. Hate it."

"What about science?"

Just stab me in the other eye. Who the fuck wants to major in these boring-ass topics?

"No. Hate that too."

"Music?" he said with some enthusiasm, hoping that I might continue his legacy.

I was getting sick of playing the trumpet and didn't want the rest of my life determined by something I wasn't sure I would like. I didn't answer and just stared at Dad.

He continued, "Art?"

My eyes lit up; my chest lightened. Maybe this was the answer.

"Art? Like finger painting?" I asked hesitantly.

"I guess," he said in an unsure tone. It was clear he didn't know much about art.

I stood there and thought for a moment. *I mean, how hard could art be?* Without giving it a second thought, I decided. "Sure. Let's do art."

Dad saw right through me and questioned my decision. "Really, what do you know about art?"

"It sounds like it's the easiest."

He let out a deep sigh, frustrated that I was not making this process easy on him or taking it seriously. "That shouldn't be the reason you pick it."

Like most teenagers, I didn't like having my logic and reasoning questioned. I crossed my arms and got right up into his face. "I don't like the other choices, and I don't even want to go to this school, so if you're going to make me go then I'm doing art."

It was settled. If I was going to have to go to a school I didn't want, then I would at least do the easiest thing there. Dad didn't argue with me. He sensed that this was more than just about picking a major. Getting up from his seat, he came over and began to rub my shoulders. In a gentle tone he told me, "You're going to be okay."

I wish I could believe you.

This was happening whether I liked it or not, and the accompanying uncertainty felt like too much to bear.

Riding the bus on my first day of school was nerve-wracking. I had a thirty-minute bus ride, including a transfer, during which my thoughts festered about all the things that could go wrong. *What if I get beaten up? Where will I sit for lunch? Are other kids on this bus going to Lane? They all look so weird. Am I dressed okay?*

As the bus pulled up to the school, I gazed upon the massive complex that was Lane Tech. *Holy shit! I don't want to do this.* I thought about taking the bus back home but knew that my mother would be there. Which was worse?

In August 1997, I walked into that building for the first time. I kept to myself that first day and tried not to draw attention. Everyone seemed to know someone with whom they went to grade school. It felt good that others were co-mingling.

Maybe the school was big enough so I could just get lost in the crowd and nobody would notice me.

At least that's what I hoped.

The person at my neighboring locker tried to approach me. He was a very chill guy who made eye contact with me. "Hey, what's your name?"

Frightened and stumbling, I got the word out: "Lenny."

"Cool," he responded and continued going about his day.

Should I have asked for his name? Oh God, get me out of here.

By third period, it was time to check out the art class. I had no idea what to expect from this major. We had assigned seats based on our last names, and I made my way over to the "G" section. The teacher started to talk about perspective, the value scale, and composition: the things we were going to study this year.

Shit! This sounded like *real* art. *What the fuck am I doing here?*

After class, I thought about changing my major to music, as my dad suggested, but it was too late. If I wanted to change my major, I was going to have to fill out a form and at the very least finish out the semester. Then there was the possibility of summer school—way too much for my anxious high school brain to deal with, amongst everything else. I guess I was going to give art a try.

Theatre fell into my lap pretty much the same way. The all-girl high school that my friends attended needed boys to audition for their upcoming fall musical. One of my girlfriends told me about it and said that I should try out. All I had to do was prepare thirty-two bars of a song, which was about thirty seconds of music.

"Come on. They are desperate for boys, and you will get cast," she told me over the phone one night.

"I don't know," I told her hesitantly, gripping the phone cord as if it were a lifeline that was somehow going to get me out of this situation.

Ignoring my reluctance, she said, "It will look good on college résumés."

How can you think about colleges as we are entering high school?

My anxiety mounted, and just to get her off the phone and avoid dealing with the situation, I said, "Fine." But soon, the doubts came in.

Me, on stage? That was a stretch. These were high school productions; this was *real* theatre. *Why did I say yes? What did I just commit to?*

I hadn't made any friends at my new school, so maybe I subconsciously said yes to be around people I knew, people who felt safe.

There was no way to get out of this. I was going to have to go through with it, so I went to my dad to ask for help in preparing my thirty-two bars. I didn't even know what to sing. Dad told me to go to his cabinet and look through all the sheet music he had stored. Scouring and searching through the cabinet, I finally came upon one song I recognized from my dad playing it on the piano.

Fuck it. It's the only number I think I can fake my way through.

We worked on it for several days, Dad coaching me as best as he could. He helped me find the correct pitch and rhythm. From my trumpet playing I knew how to read music.

On the day of the audition, I took the bus from Lane. The receptionist directed me to the auditorium where it was me, thirty to forty girls, and a handful of other boys. It was an open audition in which everyone got to watch everyone else's performance.

Oh, dear God, what did I get myself into?

I felt my chest tighten, and I held on to my sheet music as I tried to slow my breathing and not hyperventilate.

A few people went up to sing, and then . . .

"Lenny Gallo!" called out the director.

"Yes? Here!" I said. My voice cracked as I realized the full reality of what I was about to do.

"You're up!"

I got up on that huge auditorium stage and told the pianist that I would be singing "Memory" from *Cats*, a song meant for an older woman who is on the verge of death. As I heard the piano play, I took a deep breath and belted out the opening words, proclaiming the late hour of the night in my untrained voice while trying to keep my body from going into a full-blown panic attack. My eyes stared out at the audience, not sure where to direct them.

Thank God I was so naïve then about theatre, because I couldn't understand why the girls were chuckling at me when I finished, since many of them sounded like a bunch of dying cats themselves. I got cast. My friend was right. All the boys got cast. It was a small part in the ensemble.

That first semester of high school, I spent my days learning about art and my evenings doing theatre. While at first I felt unsure of these new mediums in my life, once I started to understand art and theatre, I was in heaven and couldn't get enough. I wanted to see every show that was playing in Chicago and go to every art exhibit I could. I felt genuinely connected to these dead artists, playwrights, and composers, and I wanted to know more about how they expressed themselves through these mediums. Frida Kahlo, gushing her insides out on the canvas. O'Neill telling his tales of woe in his plays. Rodgers and Hammerstein's beautiful music from *Carousel* and Andrew Lloyd Webber's *Sunset Boulevard* often blasted from my stereo. There was a sense of freedom that these visionaries had, and I wanted to feel those same things and express my thoughts, viewpoints, and feelings the way they had. I would go to the library and take out plays or books on artists, reading them intently. Or I would take out as many CDs as I could of cast albums, listening to them in my bedroom with my headphones. When I didn't understand a period or style in art or theatre, I made it my mission to study them.

Why were Rothko's blocks of color so important? And just what the hell was Beckett trying to do by burying a woman up to her neck in sand for *Happy Days*? All of them wanted to express themselves. If they could do these things, I could too. I redirected my anxious energy by creating paintings, sculptures, and drawings to explore areas of my life that I was struggling with. Or, teaching myself to channel that energy on stage, becoming someone else, forgetting that I even existed. Art and theatre provided me with a way to let out feelings of anxiety and express myself.

Art and theatre also gave me a sense of community, a sense of belonging. I wasn't the only weirdo looking to express themself. Doing shows gave me friends who were like-minded. In art class, I could connect with others who had their stories to share.

On the closing night of my very first production, I sat outside the theatre waiting for my dad to come pick me up after the cast pizza party. I looked up at the few stars you could see in the Chicago sky, took a breath of the cool, night air, and my face was beaming. As my dad's car pulled up, I jumped in with excitement.

"Did you have fun?" he asked hesitantly.

My eyes were still glowing as I thought about the whole experience of being on stage. "This is what I want to do with the rest of my life."

He smiled, nodded at me, and drove us home.

Dad would come and see every show that I was in and every school art show. He helped me practice my music and with every art project that I couldn't master on my own. There was always a smile on his face as he saw me up on stage or getting awards for my art.

My mother, on the other hand, only ever saw me on stage once and never even looked at a piece of my art. I would show her some weird thing I created, and she would turn away in disgust. Clearly, she wasn't going to be putting my stuff up on the refrigerator. The one time she came to see me in a show happened to be one of the worst days of my teenage life. One of our family dogs had just died. I woke up that morning to find him motionless in his doggy bed.

Holding back tears, worried, yet suppressing my anxiety, I turned to Mom for comfort and guidance, asking: "How am I going to go on stage today?"

She was upset about the dog, too, but it was obvious she was going to make this experience about herself. Without answering me, she ran to the phone and called my dad. She started yelling at him. I can't remember what she said, but her words seemed to insinuate, "How dare you leave me with this mess."

After she got off the phone, she frantically told me, "I can't make it today."

My sadness and anxiety shifted to anger. *What do you mean you can't make it? I can't make it in the state I'm in, but I still have to go.*

My uncle and aunt on my mother's side were also scheduled to see me in this performance. When they arrived, my aunt and uncle talked to my mother, trying to calm her down. I ignored most of the conversation with them fawning over her, but I do remember the words, "Pull yourself together. This is a big day for Len," coming out of my uncle's mouth.

I could drive myself at this point, so I headed off to the school auditorium on my own.

Before we were to go on stage, the cast sat around warming up our voices. The tears that had been building up since I found my dead dog couldn't be held in any longer. I was trying to keep it together and get through warm-ups, but a few tears dribbled down my face. The director made eye contact with me and stopped the warm-up.

"What's going on?" she asked as she approached me, her head tilted. The tears poured out as I recounted the morning's events. She embraced me and told me that everything was going to be all right. Soon some of the teenage girls and the music director came over to offer their condolences and hug me, too. It felt strange having people embrace me in my time of need: I was so used to just sucking it up and dealing with it.

Was I making too big a deal about this?

One part of it felt very right, however. The theatre had embraced me. Art had embraced me. My director and music director did something that my mother was incapable of doing—they validated my pain. It was obvious that my mother was never going to be someone I could depend on to help me with my feelings.

My mother reluctantly ended up coming. After the show, as other kids were greeting their parents and getting flowers and chocolates, I went to find my mother, aunt, and uncle. My aunt and uncle smiled at me as I came their way. They each gave me a big hug, told me how proud they were of me, and talked about how much fun it was to see me on stage.

I gazed over at my mother, who stood off in the distance. She tried not to look at me, but when our eyes met, I could see she was covering up an eternal bitterness she felt as my aunt and uncle showered me with praise.

Reflexively, I went over to her. "What did you think?" I asked, hoping for a response that, for once, showed she was happy. As she so often did in my teenage years, she answered spitefully with her usual phrase, "I never got to do these things when I was your age."

Pinching my lips tightly together, I said nothing. How do you respond to that statement? It was often her response to anything positive in my life. I always felt guilty for sharing anything positive with her, for trying to succeed, for trying to do anything better, because I knew how much it was eating her up to see me living a life that she couldn't. This guilt turned into further anxiety and continued to fuel my anger at a woman who was incapable of putting herself aside for her children. As difficult as it was, I didn't let it stop me. I turned to my art and theatre, and when I couldn't use those, I, like many other teenagers, learned very well how to bury and suppress my feelings.

Oh, and there were cigarettes: the classic prop of every great actor, writer, and artist. I took a puff of a cigarette at the age of ten, just because everyone else was doing it. At age fourteen, however, I learned how to properly inhale a cigarette. It made me nauseous, but something was alluring about the taste of smoke in my mouth and the lightheaded feeling it gave me. I knew from that moment that I was going to be a smoker. Once I learned how to smoke, how to inhale the tobacco into my lungs and hold it there, it became the single best relief for my anxiety. I have very few regrets in my life, but picking up smoking is one of them. I wish someone in my younger years had beaten this out of me, as, later in life, Edmund would dictate my ability to quit.

At age seventeen, my parents called my brother and me to the kitchen table. My dad's head hung down; my mother had an angry, bitter look on her face. "We have something to tell you," she said in an indifferent tone as she looked my brother and me in the eyes. "We're getting divorced."

Without even thinking, unfazed, I exclaimed: "Finally!"

"Oh," she muttered under her breath. "Do you have any questions?"

I sat there for a moment, trying to process what this meant. I turned to my brother, who appeared to be a little more upset than I was. Since I was the older brother, I felt he expected me to speak for both of us. There was no sadness. But that tightness in my chest began to build as I contemplated the thought that if they were getting divorced, it meant we weren't going to be living in our house. There was only one question on my mind. I looked at my father, hoping that he was not going to abandon my brother and me.

Taking a deep breath, I tried to compose myself so as not to show my hand. I put on the same fake smile my mother had often given me. "Who are we living with?" She recognized my cover-up and rolled her eyes in disgust. "You're going to live with Dad."

"But you'll see your mom on the weekends," my dad continued, looking away. He was the most hurt person in the room, but my mind wasn't there to help him that day.

Perfect. Disaster averted. The tightness in my chest released almost immediately.

And if either of you thinks I'm going to see Mom on the weekend while I've got more important shit to do with my friends, you've got another thing coming.

Anxiety always looks for safety, and my dad always did his best to make me feel safe.

My mother continued, "We'll be selling the house, and we're each going to get an apartment."

I didn't care about the details. *Do what you have to, just give me a room where I can listen to music.* As unemotionally as my mother delivered the news, I gave it right back to her: "Sounds good."

Part of me did feel an ounce of hurt, but selfishly it was more about what would happen to my brother and me. This wasn't a family. We were all existing in the same space, but everyone was doing their own thing, disconnected from each other. I was busy doing art and theatre. My brother was just about to start high school and was developing his own set of friends and ways for coping.

My mom had become embittered toward my dad, brother, and me. We weren't really a family; we never were. This was for the best.

CHAPTER 2
Scott

Toward the end of high school, my anxiety and the ensuing Edmund targeted my sexuality. It was quite stupid. Everyone knew I was gay. My mannerisms were more flamboyant, my hair color changed weekly, there were the show tunes everyone knew I loved, and my early art was certainly expressive of my sexuality. I don't know what I thought I was hiding.

Yet, I still feared how others might judge me if they *officially* knew that I liked men. I saw a mental health professional briefly to help me through this time. Slowly, I started to come out to people, and the doom and dread that I had feared about my friends judging me was not at all the way it turned out—just about everyone embraced me. We were approaching the year 2000. Ellen had come out, *Will and Grace*—all that stuff was out there. But just because a lot of my friends accepted me, it didn't mean everyone would. I couldn't just ask someone out at school; that was too risky. I knew I wanted to explore this part of myself, safely, and there was a place just for this purpose.

AOL chatrooms. The good old days. I'll save the extent of my sexual escapades on AOL for another memoir, but let's just say it was a learning experience. Much like in theatre, on AOL I could be anyone I wanted, and I took full advantage of this, getting to lead an almost double life where I could meet people who were looking to explore their sexuality. You were lucky to get a photo of the other person if they had the technology to scan it into their computer. Oftentimes, you were meeting people without any picture, just a vague description of what they might look like. Very few gay men would even consider this today. What I envisioned in my mind never matched the person in front of me when I met someone, but how else was I supposed to meet people? I find it interesting that everything else in life seemed to make me anxious, yet, without worry, I could meet men online with only an imagined picture in my brain. Perhaps feeling horny trumps anxiety. But it was through AOL that I met Scott.

Our first meeting was supposed to be a casual encounter, and I didn't tell anyone I was going to his house. My double life on AOL was very secretive; I almost felt ashamed for wanting to meet other men for sex. What made Scott different from other men I met was that we talked afterward. In fact, he wanted to talk before. He wouldn't shut the fuck up. He kept asking me all these questions, not in a perverse sort of way, but genuinely curious to get to know me. By the look on his face, I could tell that he was a caring person. This was way different from other casual encounters, where it was "Thanks for the fun night." Scott and I continued to see each other.

Scott was sweet and kind. I began to enjoy talking and getting to know him. Originally from Cleveland, Ohio, he had a melodious bass voice that he put to good use as a DJ on the radio. His voice was such a turn-on. He also had a strong, confident personality and demeanor that I found very attractive. When he walked into a room, he owned it. I wanted to know more about him and how he maneuvered through being gay. He was genuinely interested to hear about my art and theatre activities. The more we kept meeting, the more talking we would do, until one day . . .

Lying in his bed, holding each other after we had just had sex, he asked, "Do you want to go on a date sometime?" He sounded so positive about this being a good idea.

Hmmm. This is new. Does he mean go out in public?

I didn't say anything right away. He smiled at me, and I smiled back with a silly grin. I was apprehensive because, up until then, anything gay I did was done in the shadows. *Should I take this risk?* Figuring it was at least worth a try, I said: "Sure, let's go on a date."

On the night of our date, like a true gentleman, Scott picked me up. He worked for an old-school radio station at the time, and as one of their marketing gimmicks they had purchased a bunch of Volkswagen Beetles and named the cars after famous Motown artists. That night, he was driving the car named Aretha. "I remembered she's your favorite singer," he said. I couldn't stop smiling. Aretha and Madonna were my divas. Their music got me through many lonely nights.

He drove down Lakeshore Drive, heading to a trendy, novelty restaurant in downtown Chicago called the Mashed Potato Lounge. It had a club-like ambiance.

"You can put whatever you want in the mashed potatoes; they have a list of ingredients over here," Scott told me as he pointed to my menu. From the start, he was a foodie.

We were giddy at the restaurant. I put my hand on his thigh, making my way to his back to grab his ass. He smiled playfully. He took bites of my food and I of his.

As I stared into Scott's big brown eyes gleaming at me, I knew that I wanted to see him more. I had never felt like this before. My chest was loose, my stomach had a flutter, but not in an anxious way. He had won me over with pepperoni and cheddar cheese in my mashed potatoes.

Our dating life was short-lived, however. The timing wasn't right. Scott was on an upward career path, and I had just begun to figure out who I was and what I wanted to do. We weren't fully ready to commit, although we saw each other on-and-off for coffee. Each time we would meet, though, we found that same connection and spark that was there from the first time we met. As time went by, that connection grew stronger, and one day, just like that, we found ourselves deciding to be exclusive.

In college, my dream had been to major in everything to do with art and theatre. Unfortunately, I could only choose one area of study, and I selected musical theatre and honed my craft by studying voice, acting technique, and dance. In my free time over the summers, I worked on my art, and I continued with my day job waiting tables at a diner where I'd been working since I was sixteen. A local café showcased my art, and I got experience performing in local theater productions. That was probably the most exciting time in my life.

I socialized with friends I had made from grade school, high school, and beyond. We had fun at bars and went to house parties. The biggest problem we faced was . . .

"Where do you guys want to go tonight?" someone would say.

"We did that last week. Let's do this tonight and the other place tomorrow night." Everyone was getting along and having a blast. There was a sense of freedom and joy that, looking back, was all too often taken for granted.

Scott and I were also in a great place. One of the fringe benefits of dating someone who worked in radio was that he could always get us tickets to the latest concert in town.

"You got tickets to Madonna? I love you!" I told him playfully.

"You'd better," he would say playfully back.

We would go out for dinner, and he introduced me to cuisines I had never experienced: Indian, sushi. What the hell were these things? I loved it. Unfortunately, years later, after trying lobster with Scott, I would learn of a seafood allergy that could kill me. But it was fun while it lasted.

My anxiety and worry were pretty much under control, and everything felt very right. But it didn't take long for it to come back. Scott got a job offer that would take him to Los Angeles.

When he told me, I became frenzied, got in my car, and blew through stop signs as I drove to his place with the hope that he would have a solution to this problem he had just presented. At this point, I had been given a key to his apartment, and let myself in. I opened the door. He was on the phone telling a friend about his job offer. He turned to look at me and saw that I was trying not to cry. As he ended his call, I ran to hug him. "I don't want you to go," I mumbled.

Scott took me in his arms, squeezed me tight, and said, "I don't know what this means for us."

My eyes widened. *You don't have a plan? You would just leave me for this fucking job?*

Hurt and somewhat confused, I hid my thoughts and feelings, but I wanted to hit him and scream at him. *Wasn't I enough for him?*

My mind started to fixate on thoughts that I did not like. Scott was one of the few gay men I had ever been able to connect with on a deep level, and I didn't want to give that up. We spent the whole night talking, reflecting on how far our relationship had come, saying what we wanted for our futures. The reality was that I had to finish school, and he had to take this job. We decided to give a long-distance relationship a try and see what would happen.

My anxiety resurfaced, strongly.

In my final years of college, I got cast in shows in Chicago—nothing much, but enough to build my résumé. After Scott had moved to L.A., I visited during breaks and summer. He showed me all the fun spots, but it didn't take long to realize that I was not happy out there. L.A. was like one giant suburb, and I didn't see the appeal. The houses were all pinks, yellows, and pastels. Everything was so bright. Who the hell would want to live in that? Yes, Los Angeles had film, but I was a stage actor. All the greats got their start on Broadway.

How do I tell him I don't want to live out here?

Guilt overtook me for even having these thoughts. Torn about how to reconcile my feelings for Scott but not wanting to live in Los Angeles, I pretended everything was okay. Deep down inside, however, I knew it would not work. I didn't think Scott and I were going to make it much past this.

Fate again intervened. It just so happened that Scott's Los Angeles job was short-lived, but he found another one almost immediately: a job that would enable him to move to market number one—New York City. This changed the equation. Broadway was my dream.

Scott didn't want to leave Los Angeles; he loved it out there. But this job gave him a once-in-a-lifetime opportunity that he couldn't pass up. He took the job. I was relieved and happy that I didn't have to tell him I wouldn't be joining him in Los Angeles if he stayed.

When Scott moved to the East Coast, he initially got an apartment in Hoboken, New Jersey, just across the river from Manhattan. I visited him several times before finishing school. These were some of my happiest memories with him. It was like we were dating again. We had a ton of fun seeing shows; getting to really explore the city. As graduation day approached, Scott started to think about us reconnecting on a more permanent level.

The weird thing about a long-distance relationship was that when we got together, we knew it was temporary, so we tried to make the most of the time. I could go back to my life, and he to his. But now we were talking about joining these lives together. The stars had aligned, but this decision prompted even further anxiety.

There were a tremendous number of trepidations I had about moving from Chicago to New York, even though I wanted to live there. I loved Scott, but now other questions tore at me:

Was I ready to make such a big move on my own? Was I prepared to give up my life in Chicago? It had taken me so long to build a comfortable life where I had friends and was doing what I wanted. Did I really want to lose that?

With the new money Scott was making from his job, he decided it was time to buy a house. "You're going to love it. It's a unique property," he would say enthusiastically as we talked on the phone.

A house? I thought, rather terrified. What was I doing? New York? How do I even navigate that? In Chicago, I knew where I stood. In New York, I would have to start from scratch.

"What am I going to do for work?" I asked him.

"Stop worrying. We're going to be fine. There's tons of jobs waiting tables out here. You want to be out here, right?"

"Absolutely," I told him, secretly thinking, *I'm not sure*. This was a huge decision to make.

Scott never really understood my fears about moving. Being in radio, he moved constantly. This was just another city he had to move to. For me, this was a complete uprooting of my life.

I spent days and weeks ruminating on the decision. My mind never stopped spinning and I leaned on my friends for guidance.

"What do I do? Do I move in with Scott? Do I move out east? Do I want to be in a different time zone? I like Central Time," I would say, hoping that one of them would come up with a piece of information I hadn't already pondered.

They gave me all sorts of different answers. I didn't know whose opinions to trust, and I sure couldn't trust myself. Anxiety doesn't allow you to trust yourself. This all felt so weird and uncertain. Nobody could tell me how to make this decision. It was mine alone.

One friend did suggest something I hadn't considered: "This can just be a test; you can always move back if you want."

That felt safe-ish. I needed to know that I could back out at any time. My twenty-three-year-old brain was able to process that. With my belongings packed, it was time to head to New York.

The day of my move everyone came to see me off—my dad, my friends. Even my mother made an appearance, but it was less about me leaving and more about her curiosity as to how my dad was doing since their divorce. My chest was so constricted, I could barely breathe as I packed the last of my stuff into the van. I hugged everyone, and kissed Chicago goodbye. Scott had flown out to make the fourteen-hour drive back east with me. While Scott and I were driving down 80-East, I spent the better part of it crying, thinking to myself, *This is just a test. This is just a test.*

I had not yet seen the house that Scott had bought, so I had no idea where he was taking me. We crossed the northeastern state line of New Jersey and wound our way on the roads of what would soon be my new neighborhood. It all felt so quiet and isolated.

"Are we out in the country?" I asked Scott as we pulled up to the house.

"No, it's a suburb," he said, laughing at me. "We're fifteen miles away from the city." Something didn't seem right about this. There were a bunch of mixed emotions that I was experiencing, and I was not sure of how to verbalize them. I smiled politely.

Living in the burbs was a culture shock from growing up in a city. You had to drive everywhere. The public transportation was horrendous in Jersey. I had given up my car, thinking I wouldn't need it, and hadn't planned on being so far away from New York. In Chicago, you drove, but you could also walk down the block for anything you needed or take the train. Everything out here was far apart from everything else, and it was so family-friendly. Where were the gays? Where was the culture? To keep my feelings in check, I would repeat my mantra: "This is just a test. You can always go back."

The initial shock lessened, and it was time to go forth to pursue my career.

Auditioning in New York was much different from auditioning in Chicago. In a smaller market like Chicago, I felt like I had a chance to at least be seen and show others what I could do. New York had a lot of young, aspiring actors and was about cattle call auditions. If you didn't get your name on that list by 6:00 a.m. and try to be one of the first fifty people on that sheet, there was a good chance you weren't getting seen for the day. Three to five times a week, I would stand at the bus stop from Jersey to New York and spent entire days at studios hoping to be seen.

I waited one such day at one of the big three audition studios for a production of *Annie*. After six hours, my name was called. Walking into the small room where the production staff sat, I clenched my music book, trying to channel my anxiety through my tight fists.

Auditioning was such an anxiety-inducing process. Even though I had done it dozens of times, it never got easier. You never knew what they were looking for from you. I followed standard protocol and walked over to the pianist with my book of music and had a brief conversation about what song I would sing.

"Tonight at Eight," I told him as I flipped through my music book. My sheet music was always meticulously organized and highlighted to make it easy for the pianist. Ready to begin, I stood there waiting for them to cue me. No one looked up. I expected someone on the casting team to give me a nod or ask me a question, but no one did. I turned to the pianist, who nodded his head and started to play.

As was often the case during auditions, I felt my heart pounding as I started to sing. Once I began, though, it was as if a spirit had taken over me. My nerves settled, and I became another character.

You never are supposed to look at casting staff—every actor knows that—but as I finished belting my last note, my eyes gazed their way. Not a single person had looked up. They were eating their lunch, playing on their phones, and doing God knows what. I finished and looked back at the pianist, who was already closing my book and handing it to me.

I waited a moment longer. Generally, at the end of an audition, they would at least say "thank you." Even if they did not like you, they said thank you as a courtesy, which cued you to leave the room. But on that day, in that room, it was as if I didn't exist. Not sure of what to do, I stood there for a few moments before walking to the exit.

Not even a thank you? I thought to myself as I walked out of the room, drained from a six-hour day of sitting around waiting to be seen for what ended up being all of thirty seconds.

Trying to be mindful of careless mistakes that could be avoided, on the bus ride home to Jersey, I always wrote a self-critique in my audition journal as a way of learning for the next audition. *What to put for this* one? It was as if I was a ghost who had just floated in and out of that room with no one the wiser that I had even been there.

Am I really cut out for this? I wondered, jerking my head up as it fell toward my chest, trying not to fall asleep as the bus drove through the Lincoln Tunnel.

Money was running low for me, and it was clear I needed to get a job. Scott was helping me financially, but I didn't want him to think I was a freeloader, and I did want to take care of myself. Initially, I planned to get a job waiting tables in New York. Many places required headshots, however, and if you didn't look the part, you weren't getting hired. Even Scott was baffled by this.

"They want headshots? For serving food?" he asked, as we looked at some of the ads. "Is that legal?"

They also wanted you to already have experience at a New York restaurant. Most people just lied, but my Midwestern ethical values made me worry about what would happen if they called the restaurant I put down as a reference. I couldn't chance it and ended up settling. I took a job at a chain restaurant five miles down the road from where we lived. It was fancier than the diner I had worked at in Chicago, but it was the same bullshit of waiting tables. Not having a car, I had to take the bus on days Scott could not drive me, and what would have been a ten-minute car trip turned into a two-hour bus ride. This added to my frustration: getting around and being independent were predicated on an unreliable bus schedule.

What the fuck am I doing out here? I would think, angry that I didn't have my independence. My anxiety escalated as I tried to navigate through all these changes. *Why did I move out here? Am I in the right career? Do I even want to be with Scott?* Daily, my brain would rummage around to figure out ways to make this work, but I was young and didn't have a lot of guidance. These weren't easy questions to answer.

I didn't feel comfortable talking to Scott about how I felt; he was trying so hard to build a life for us. I turned to my friends in Chicago.

Calling them became part of my daily routine and a comfort. I told them of my unhappiness and how confused I was. They offered their support as best as they could. The one thing I knew for sure, this was too much change for me. After only nine months, I decided it was time to go back home.

I didn't have the heart to share my real feelings with Scott. I'm not proud of this, but I lied to him and told him I had been cast in a show back in Chicago. I did end up getting an offer, but I wasn't going to take it. I was just looking for an excuse to get out. The constant anxiety was too much, and I wasn't sure I was ready for all of these major life changes hitting me all at once. I wanted to go back to the security of what I knew. Scott was devastated when I broke the news.

Before I drove off with all of my stuff in a rented truck, I hugged Scott goodbye for what might have been forever. He hugged me and sobbed. "I hope this isn't the last time I see you."

It was a Monday morning when I reprised my role as a diner waiter in Chicago. I put on my apron, and it was as if I had never left. Customers that I had waited on a year prior were still coming. Now I had to answer all the questions.

"Why are you back? What happened?" they asked, not out of concern, but to see if they could get the latest gossip to fuel their boring lives.

As I waited on tables that day, carrying scrambled eggs and bacon to the blue-collar working class that patronized the restaurant, I felt another sense of dread.

What did I just do? I had made a life-altering decision and had given up a lot for the two and three-dollar tips I was getting. This feeling of dread grew even deeper when I started to reconnect with my friends. In the nine months I had been gone, so much had changed with them. It was as if I was walking into a world that had been flipped upside down. Some were getting married and having children. New people had entered friend groups, and I felt so out of place.

As I scrounged change together to cover my rent, I was devastated to receive phone calls from shows that I had auditioned for months prior back in New York. They wanted to cast me, but now it was too late. Had I underestimated myself?

And Scott, I found myself missing him, missing the life we were creating, and missing the opportunity to give it my all with theatre and art. Scott and I talked on the phone daily, and eventually I fessed up about why I left. He was hurt, but a part of him understood. He said he appreciated my honesty and wanted me to work through my issues, but he also wanted a partner. If I wasn't coming back, he wanted to move on with his life.

Scott and I spent many nights talking about what went wrong when I came out to New Jersey. A part of me knew that Chicago wasn't the answer, and I needed to reassess. We agreed that we loved each other and wanted to be with each other, but some things would have to change if I was going to move back and we were going to give it another try.

For starters, I needed to get some rock ballads and more contemporary music under my belt. Theatre was changing, and I wasn't keeping up with the trend. I decided to refine my craft by going back to my voice teachers, learning from my mistakes. It was also clear that I was not going to spend the rest of my life waiting tables. I needed a better day job. While I was still back in Chicago, I decided to go for something that had always been in the back of my mind. I loved getting massages, and after talking to people in the field, becoming a massage therapist seemed like a perfect fit for me. They apparently made decent money, and I'd much rather do that than serve tables while waiting for my big break. At night, I studied the anatomy of the human body and how to properly touch it.

During this time, I started journaling and began to imagine a world where I could create stories. I read all the books I could on how to construct plays and scripts, and I vowed that once I was back in New York I would take classes to learn this new craft.

Most importantly, I decided that I needed a car. If I was going to live in Jersey, a car was a must. My great aunt had recently passed and left me a little bit of money. New car. Check.

After working through what I thought were all my issues, Scott and I set a move-in date. I again packed up my things and headed back to the East Coast. No fancy sendoff this time, just me putting whatever I could bring in my little car and heading back out. This time, I felt ready to take on this challenge. But my anxiety was relentless and latched on to whatever wasn't perfect. And it would continue to feed Edmund's eventual growth.

Empty Inside, 2012, oil on canvas, 4" x 4".

CHAPTER 3
Empty Inside

Scott and I were sitting in a coffee shop once I was back in New Jersey, me with my copy of *Backstage*, the actors' weekly trade paper. Three weeks back, I hit the ground running and browsed every page of each issue, circling any parts I thought I was good for— and even parts I probably wasn't suited for. I was determined to not let fear and anxiety hold me back from auditioning, so I tucked those feelings away in a place that only I could find.

I took a sip of my latte and told Scott excitedly, "Look, a cruise line is auditioning. I heard this was an easy way to get your equity card." Your equity card meant getting a chance to actually be able to audition for Broadway. Without it, you'd never be seen.

He looked at me, angry and confused. "How long would that be?"

"It says thirteen months, plus it could get me my equity card."

He said, "You just got here. You would really go off and leave again?"

I could tell by his tone he wasn't happy with the idea of me leaving when we had already been apart for so long. But didn't he understand the life of actors? You took what work was available. Plus, he moved plenty of times for his career. This was a cruise ship for thirteen months.

"I could always audition just for the hell of it, see what happens . . . I mean, it's not like I'm going to get it."

Guilting me, he asked, "You'd really tempt fate?"

Conflicted and angry, I wasn't quite sure how to respond. I tucked that angry feeling away and said, "You're probably right."

Maybe he was right. Did I really want to leave having just moved here? A part of me wanted to try. A little voice told me to go for it. But I didn't know how to say that to him. I didn't listen to that voice. I used logic, instead, to get me through this one. He *was* right. We had been apart for a long time. Maybe now wasn't the time for something like this. My searches were kept to local stuff in the tri-state area. I pushed through all my fears, and within a couple of months I was getting cast. Every part I was offered, I took. It didn't matter what it was, local theater in Jersey, children's theatre in Long Island, New York workshops, off-off Broadway, I did it all.

I still remember the moment I felt I had made it as an actor. *The Majestic Theatre*, housed on 45th Street and 8th Avenue, had one of the longest-running shows on Broadway, *Phantom of the Opera*. Down the block, closer to 9th Avenue, was a tiny space where I was performing in an off-off Broadway workshop. When I walked outside during breaks, I crossed the street and looked *way* down the block, where you could barely see the Phantom's white mask that adorned the theatre marquis for so many years. Being that close to such an iconic show took me back to the feelings of pure bliss that I had the night I closed my very first high school show. I stared at that sign with such optimism every time I walked outside. It was the closest I have ever felt to my dreams.

Auditioning for shows took up so much of my time, I didn't create much art then, but I never let that part of me go and managed to create a few pieces here and there when the moment felt right. It was nothing much, but it was something.

My first day at a popular massage chain couldn't come fast enough.

I was once again on the brink of running out of money. It took me three months to get hired. In the burbs of Jersey, male massage therapists were not as popular as our female counterparts. Men didn't want men touching them, and women didn't want to be naked in a room with a man. I wanted to work in New York, but this time it was fucking licensing requirements that wouldn't allow my Illinois license to transfer; something I hadn't counted on. The massage chain was the only place in Jersey willing to take a chance on me.

That first day, I had five people scheduled. My boss told me, "The goal is to get one person to sign up for a membership." In Chicago, my training required an extensive program: one thousand hours versus the three hundred hours required out here in New Jersey; I felt confident I could deliver. "Piece of cake."

I gave probably five of the best massages I have ever given, and every single person signed up for a membership. As I was walking out, my boss smiled at me, while the other employees looked at me dumbfounded. Soon, I became one of the most requested therapists.

To improve my writing, I joined a playwriting group and was desperately trying to finish a full-length play. An idea I had for a show seemed like a great concept. It kept spinning around in my head, and I wanted to see that idea through to fruition. My writers' group was a great outlet for me. I would bounce ideas off other individuals, hear them read my script, and I enjoyed every moment of it.

Around this time, I met Nick, an older man who ended up casting me in an independent film he was directing. He had a very strong New Jersey accent and the thickest dark brown hair I had ever seen. We went to lunch one afternoon a few months after shooting the film.

"I'm going to be casting for an upcoming musical workshop . . . It's nothing big, but I think you would be good for one of the parts."

Without hesitation, I gave a resounding, "Yes."

During this lunch, I learned that he was a writer as well. Nick also followed every ounce of what was happening on Broadway and was a theatre queen like me. Unlike many others that I came in contact with, he also lived out in Jersey. Most people I met in the acting world were based in New York. It was nice to have someone else who was local. He cast me in the show, and through that process we became friends. When the show closed, we were both determined to focus on finishing pieces we were writing, and we spent hours going over our writing on the phone.

"I just finished a scene; I'm sending it to you now," Nick would say enthusiastically.

"It's shit. Try it this way," I would say to him, confident that I was right. He would take my feedback and go with it.

He did the same for me, too. "No, this isn't working, cut it, it's shit."

It felt good to have a writing buddy and connect with someone like-minded. There wasn't a day that went by when we didn't talk at least once. Things appeared to be moving in the right direction.

For the next five years, I was doing my best to make my way on the East Coast, and I put everything I had into my craft. I buried all my fears and trepidations and tried to pave a path for myself—but you can't bury your fears and trepidations forever.

My massage career was going well, but the massage industry was changing. I got into the business right on the cusp of this change but was too naïve to notice. Massage therapists were forced to take big pay cuts. The industry used to be a place where you could see ten to twelve people a week and easily make $150 per massage. Now, with the discount massage chains slowly taking over, you made closer to $20 a massage plus tip. My job at one of these chains was supposed to be a starting point, but other massage places were closing, because they couldn't keep up with the competitive prices. This meant I would have to hold onto this job, which required seeing many more people and working longer hours. I wasn't making the money I had hoped for, and it left me feeling very dependent on Scott.

Stress and anxiety would ensue when I got sick and had to take a day off, because this would affect my finances. Snow days, while fun when you are a kid, could mean losing hundreds of dollars. The first time I noticed a pain in my wrist that couldn't be stretched out caused me a bit of alarm.

I was fed up with always having to work odd hours and shifts to pay the bills. For my whole work life, I had been a manual laborer and puppeteer for someone else's pleasure. The unsustainability of this career consumed my thoughts.

Why was money such a concern? Anyone who's ever attempted to make a living in the arts knows you rarely make any money. Yes, many people do make a great living in the arts, but not early on in your career and not nearly enough. It's not just actors: writers, artists, musicians, and others often are expected to work for free or basically for free much of the time, just for the chance to get another credit on one's résumé or the experience.

Acting was also starting to take a toll on me. I'll admit, my definition of success was skewed. If I didn't make it on Broadway, win a Tony, *and* have a play that was running for years, then I was a failure.

I had just closed in a production of the Revolutionary War-themed musical *1776* at a children's theatre. The children we performed for were acting silly, rolled their eyes in boredom, and ultimately hurled Skittles at us. When I practiced my Tony Award-winning speech as a teenager in my bedroom, getting candy thrown at me wasn't part of the process and not exactly what I had in mind when I initially set out for my New York Adventure. I was becoming very disillusioned by the business.

Many times, I was cast in a show simply because I was the only person available to do the part. This is a great way to break in at first, but it seemed to get old after a while. I could never really land the parts I wanted.

I'm a short man in a character actor's body with a classically trained tenor voice. People would often compliment the tone and pitch of my "beautiful" lyric sound. But it was hard for me to find my type. An acting teacher back in college once told me: "I might cast you as an elf, or a leprechaun."

I was gay, but not gay enough for the parts at the time. I could pull off straight, so long as I wasn't the love interest. If I was going to be cast as the love interest, which I could pull off vocally, my leading lady had to be shorter than me.

My worst time as an actor was during a show for a new work. I tried for weeks to find my character's intention, motivation, and reasons for doing things, pissing off the writer and director in the process. I realized that my part could have, and should have, been cut from the show completely. Every night, I had to get up on a stage and try to sell myself in this part, only to watch the audience squirming in their seats and looking at their watches for how much longer they had to endure this torture.

I tried to have fun with every part I was given and make it my own, put my own spin on it, and lose myself in the role. But it seemed like there was no space for someone like me and that I would have to take whatever table scraps were thrown my way. The business was making me very bitter. What once was a lifeline for creative expression now was just like any other job that seemed thankless.

Things only got worse when it came to my writing. I wrote myself into walls, unable to solve storylines and structural problems with my manuscripts. I was driving Scott, Nick, and my playwriting group crazy.

"Just try it like this," Nick would say to me on the phone, trying to help me work through things.

"No, that's not going to work either."

"What about doing it this way?"

Fuck that. You don't know what you're talking about.

In my writing workshop I got the words no writer ever wants to hear: "Maybe you need to take a break from this piece."

No! Never! I can't let this die.

"Yeah, maybe," I said, as the thought of failure invaded my mind, and I watched something that felt so right be torn apart. To this day, if I even mention the name of that play to anyone who was around me at that time, they cringe. I must have traumatized everyone with my incessant need for feedback on a story that just wasn't working.

And my art, my painting. I couldn't find anything that would inspire me. Worry consumed me as I questioned what my future would look like.

All of this felt like I was going nowhere. I was terribly unhappy with the arts. While I loved acting and singing on stage, writing, and painting, I was burning out, and it wasn't offering me much in the way of a payoff.

Probably the biggest problem during this time was my relationship with Scott. The age difference was rarely a factor except with a little teasing from our friends. Around this time, however, it was very clear that we were in two different places in our lives and careers. Scott had the luxury of working at home, was able to quit working for radio stations and make his living as a freelance voiceover artist. I, on the other hand, was massaging people's feet, scrounging money to cover my share of the bills. Living with Scott was also quite different from dating Scott.

When I first moved out here, everything was so new I hadn't given much thought to what it would be like to live with someone long-term. But after years of living with him now, I started to see a different side; stuff that I had noticed, but never gave much thought to. He was stubborn, set in his ways, and was incredibly particular about food. I always tried to put fun toys and trinkets around the house, but whenever I did, he would respond in a disparaging tone, "This doesn't work with our décor."

Fuck the décor! Isn't this my place, too? I thought, angrily holding back my feelings.

Somewhere in this process, I had inadvertently settled into the role of housewife without even realizing it. I would make sure to clean and make dinners. On Tuesday mornings, I would give it my best shot with my downward-facing dog in a yoga class that consisted of me and twenty soccer moms who had the morning free from the kids. And, like any good housewife, I felt unappreciated.

As he was drying himself after a shower, I asked Scott, "Why do you have to use a new towel every day?"

"Because I'm not putting a dirty towel on my face that had been on my ass. What does it matter?"

"Because I'm the one who washes the towels. Your ass should be clean after you shower. And the dishes go *in* the dishwasher."

These petty issues arose from deeper-rooted ones within me. When I looked at Scott, I didn't see the man I once fell in love with. I blamed him for things that were going wrong in my life. He was paying the majority of the bills and paying for the house, which made me feel trapped and like I could never express my true feelings about our relationship. When I tried to bring my feelings up, Scott would try and debate me rather than listen. I began to loathe being in his presence.

"What do you want for dinner?" he would ask as we sat in the car.

Does it really matter what I want? You're just going to say no, I thought to myself as I sat there next to him.

Breathing out my anxiety and frustration, I would say with a blank look on my face, "Whatever, doesn't matter."

In a genuinely sincere tone, he would say, "I picked last time. What do you want?"

I offered my suggestion, but I knew where this was going. "How about the diner?"

Instantly dismissing the idea, he responded, "They're overpriced, and their food is awful. Where else?"

A little more frustrated, I tried to offer another suggestion. "White . . .?"

Sarcastically, he responded and cut me off before I could get the words out, ". . . Really, fast food?"

Fast food wasn't good for you or the best option, I knew that. But I grew up on the stuff, and there was always some comfort from the evil corporate entities making America fat. I didn't like conflict; if this conversation went any further, one would certainly ensue. I put on my usual fake smile to avoid it and told him, "Whatever you want."

Scott's strong personality, which initially attracted me to him, didn't make it easy to communicate with him. It was both a blessing and a curse. He was assertive when he needed to be, but sometimes his assertiveness was misconstrued.

A friend of mine was visiting once, and we were all riding in Scott's car. Like he did so many other times, Scott would scream and yell at every asshole driver on the road. "What the fuck are you doing?" he would shout at the other car as he laid on the horn, trying to tailgate them and show them how much of an asshole they were being. In his defense, the drivers on the East Coast were quite nightmarish.

Later, when my friend and I were alone, she asked me in a rather serious tone. "Does he beat you?"

I laughed, thinking she was joking. "Oh, God, No."

"He just seems to get very angry very quickly," she pointed out, still somewhat concerned.

"He's always like that when he drives," I responded. I was used to this behavior, but if a person didn't know Scott very well, I could see how they might interpret him in this way.

Scott didn't scare me, but what did were the questions I started asking about him.

Why would he buy a house in the suburbs without even considering me?
Why did he guilt me into not auditioning for tours?
What the fuck is with the towels?
Why don't I get a say with dinners?

Even scarier than the questions was the bitterness I started to notice within me, imagining that this was what my mother felt like toward my father. I had prided myself on never repeating my mother's behavior, but when it came to my relationship . . . *Am I becoming my mother?*

This thought scared the crap out of me, because I never wanted to become someone that I associated with so much anger.

Rarely would I share my feelings about my life with anyone. I thought: *Was I too entitled? Was I making too big a deal about all of this?*

My art, my acting, my writing, and my relationship—everything in my life seemed to be coming to a head in my late twenties, and I had no idea how to fix any of it. Anxiety and worry provoked daily panic attacks. I would sit outside on the balcony of our house, questioning what the next steps would be, but the more I deliberated, the emptier I became. All my attempts to solve the problems were leaving me with additional questions that had no real answers.

And I was alone in New Jersey. I started closing myself off from the world. Often, I would talk to my friends in Chicago, trying to get support. When I spoke to them, however, and heard tales of their accelerating careers, I questioned what I was doing in life. They all seemed to be building lives while I was stuck in this weird limbo. If I wasn't an artist or an actor anymore, then what was I? If I didn't love Scott, then what would happen? I reflected on my entire life up until now and found no way of reconciling my decisions, my feelings, and my behavior. Now it wasn't just anxiety I was dealing with; it was depression as well. This feeling became so intense that I finally thought it was time to see somebody.

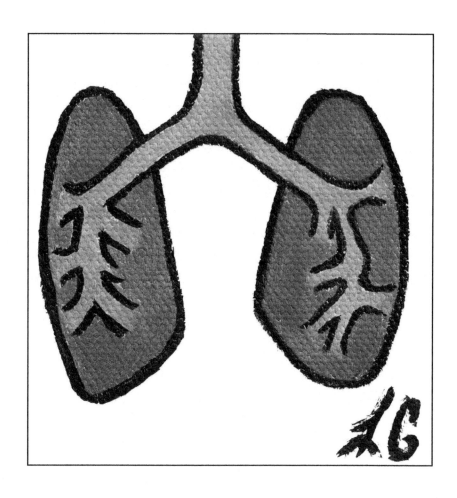

Anxiety, 2012, oil on canvas, 3" x 3".

CHAPTER 4

"Am I Going To Die?!"

There is usually a whole set of physiological symptoms that manifest from anxiety and depression and cannot be explained by any medical tests or doctors. I would get unexplained headaches and migraines, my head was constantly spinning, and the worst one was that my stomach was always a mess. Constantly, I ruminated about my health. Feeling miserable most of the time and never knowing what to do or what to eat, I tried to push through all these symptoms. Crackers, breads, rice, and ginger ale became my friends. Scott had the stomach of an iron pit. Nothing bothered him, and not being able to eat certain foods was a foreign concept to him. He tried to be supportive, but he never entirely understood what it meant to not be able to enjoy food.

Stomach issues are common among those with anxiety. Throughout most of my early and mid-twenties, I was plagued with gastroesophageal reflux disease and digestive discomfort, but normally it was manageable. It started to grow increasingly worse, and I found no real relief in the usual solutions of bismuth and other over-the-counter stomach aids.

My first trip to a doctor to manage my mental health was to a gastro-enterologist. Rather than deal with the real issues that underscored my anxiety, I deemed it more important to ignore the problems and keep pushing forward.

Dr. Pelkington, a gastroenterologist located in Mahwah, New Jersey, had a small office in a medical complex. After I signed in, paid my copay, and filled out his mounds of paperwork, he finally saw me. He did what seemed like a basic examination and tried to make small talk.

"What do you do for work?" he asked as he rubbed my bloated belly.

Trying not to pass gas as he dug deeper, I said, "I'm an actor . . . and a massage therapist." I learned long ago that if I just said actor, people would give me a look that implied: *Really? What's your day job?* Honestly, I always felt a sense of shame just saying actor. Who the hell was I? I wasn't DeNiro or Brando.

Dr. Pelkington checked my blood pressure and neck. He put his stethoscope on my stomach and back. He even gave me my first prostate exam/massage, put a drop of petroleum jelly on his latex-covered index finger, and shoved it into my anus. *Not enough lube, Dr. Pelkington . . . not enough lube.*

Dr. Pelkington couldn't provide answers, but he definitely added to my anxiety.

"This could be a lot of things. We're going to have to run some tests."

Tests? Okay, I can handle tests. That's why I came to you, I thought, feeling confident that some blood work could get to the bottom of what was going on.

I noticed that he was writing what seemed to be lengthy notes.

Why is he writing so much?

Curious, I forced myself to whisper, "What could this be?"

Not even taking his eyes off his prescription pad, he said in a very dry tone, "It could be a brain tumor, or diverticulitis, colon cancer . . . It's hard to say."

It took a moment to register what he had said, but then my heart sank to my stomach, and I could feel my chest tighten up.

Tumor? Cancer? Holy shit! I'm going to die.

My mind raced a mile a minute. Hearing those words brought a sense of terror that almost set off a panic attack.

"I'm ordering a CAT scan of your brain and some other tests."

Am I going to die?! From this stomach issue?! I sat for a moment, plotting out how I was going to tell my dad and Scott that we needed to start making funeral arrangements. All the big questions started coming into my brain, and the sense of my impending death dominated the next couple of weeks of my life.

Dr. Pelkington put me into debt by running a multitude of tests that would rule out anything major. Everything was on the table, from a tumor to hemorrhoids.

Anxiety 101: You can't tell an anxious person that they might have a tumor. When someone says tumor, you must get the test. You can't not get the test. It's scarier not to know, and I had no choice but to follow up on this and all the tests he ordered. Sure enough, several weeks later . . .

He stared at the results of the CAT scan of my brain for all of ten seconds before proceeding to tell me jokingly, in an awful impression of Arnold Schwarzenegger, "It's not a tumor."

"Ha-ha . . . very good," I said with a fake stage laugh. I breathed deeply for what seemed to be my first breath in the ten days leading up to the results of this test. The only thought running through my brain in that moment, however, was *You piece of shit. Do you have any idea how torturous this has been?* I wanted to kill this man for the mental anguish he inflicted on me, but, since I needed him to tell me what was *actually* going on, I said nothing.

None of the other tests revealed anything either: shitting in a cup and gathering my feces daily for assessment; blood work and rectal exams. Ironically, everything but a colonoscopy or endoscopy, which I didn't think to even question at the time. The final verdict: "This sounds like IBS."

After costing me five thousand dollars, he told me I had irritable bowel syndrome and said, "Maybe we should take an all-natural approach."

Really, that wasn't a first step? All natural comes after you order a CAT scan of my head and have me rummage through my feces? I wanted to slam this man into a wall.

Breathe, I though to myself. This man is here to help you. "Sure, let's try all-natural," I said.

He told me I could get regular colon cleansings, which can sometimes reset the peristalsis or the movement in the GI tract. He told me about all the right foods to eat and exercises I could do. I tried all of this for several months. When nothing helped, I went back and reported my findings. It was then that he introduced me to a pill that was "better than the over-the-counter medications" I was taking. "I'm going to prescribe something. This should help with all your symptoms," he said, writing on his prescription pad.

It was exciting to think that there might be something that might help me with all my stomach issues. I was always pro-pill and never had a problem taking medication. But as any good patient would do, I asked: "Any side effects?"

"Nothing to worry about. You can take this as needed up to three times a day."

Reglan, generically known as metoclopramide, was my first intro to medications that can affect your brain chemistry. It would be the sperm of Edmund that would get impregnated in me, but at the time that was an unknown. Reglan was amazing. Never did a pill help me more in life than this little guy.

Acid Reflux? Reglan's got you. Constipated? Reglan's got that, too. Feeling nauseous? You betcha—your good friends at the pharmaceutical companies put Reglan on the market to help with that, too. It was the best thing out there, and I took it as often as I needed.

I got to the point where I didn't have to see Dr. Pelkington anymore and just got a prescription from my general practitioner. Around that time, though, I realized that my anxiety was becoming more agitated. I couldn't quite explain it, but I felt like I had a ton of nervous energy that needed to get out. My body always had to do something to keep me busy, but I attributed this anxious energy to events at the time and a general sense that I was not happy with the direction that my life was going. Reglan might have been helping my stomach, but my anxiety and depression were becoming more paralyzing.

"Honey, what's wrong?" Scott often asked as we sat at the dining room table for dinner. I would bust out crying: "I don't know," I would say as I spit out bits of food, not knowing how to verbalize all the thoughts in my mind. "Everything. Everything is wrong."

"Try and cheer up," he would say, with a look of sorrow on his face.

Cheer up? You have no idea what's going on inside of me. My negative feelings about Scott continued to build. Couldn't he see that everything was wrong? It wasn't just Scott, but my writing, my acting, my art. What was I doing with my life?

Scott tried to understand, but he never really grasped the concept of mental health. Depression and anxiety weren't part of his vocabulary. Feeling like things weren't going your way didn't resonate with him. He grew up with a different set of values.

The couch became my friend, and binge-watching TV was my thing now. Luckily, Nick was a TV fanatic as well, and he was able to make recommendations. I would often talk to him about my anxiety and feelings, and he tried to cheerlead me through them. "You need to stop being Norma Desmond. Stop being a drama queen. The more you give in to this depression, the more it's going to take you down."

Depression is an awful feeling; it sucks you into a hole. Scott wasn't trying to be insensitive, and Nick wasn't trying to minimize my depression. A lot of people don't know what to say to people when they're depressed or anxious. They tried to get me out of it as best as they knew how, and I felt like I was doing everything I could to keep my anxiety and depression under control. But when the stomach issues intensified, the energy of the anxiety increased, the depression hit me at my core, and I finally had enough of the days spent on the couch watching TV; I broke down and decided it was time to see a mental health professional—a psychiatrist.

CHAPTER 5
Do Not Knock

I didn't know what to make of psychiatrists. The only experience I had with them was connected to my mother, and they didn't seem to work for her. Attempting to find a psychiatrist can be a challenge, especially finding one in-network with your insurance. My options were very limited, and the wait times were ridiculous.

"The soonest he could see you would be in three months," a receptionist would say very coldly on the phone.

"Sorry, we're not taking new patients right now," said another in the same tone.

Then why does it say online that you are?

After weeks of calling places, I eventually came across a woman who had been in the business for years. I equated time in the business with being good, and I took her next available appointment, one month away.

Dr. Baldisseri was an older woman who ran her own practice out of a rented studio space in Fairfield, New Jersey. I was very excited the first time I pulled up to her office because it was clear that there was a lot on my mind that needed to come out. I just needed a venue in which to express myself.

I walked into the office complex, scanned the office directory posted at the entrance, found her name, and made my way up to the second floor. The office was in a multipurpose, dingy, older building. There were law offices, psychiatrists, and other professionals who shared a communal waiting room. Outside her door were two chairs. A clipboard said: "Please sign in. Dr. Baldisseri will come out to get you. Do not knock on door!!!"

Not the most inviting clipboard, but okay, I thought, trying not to prejudge her.

I put my name on the paper and took a seat. I was incredibly nervous and excited at the same time. I was finally going to get to the bottom of this anxiety and depression and learn ways to cope and deal with it. I thought about all the things I was going to tell her: my struggles with my play, my difficulties in my relationship, trying to figure out the next steps for my life. I was ready.

An hour passed and there was still no sign of her.

I started to lose my motivation to talk. My initial excitement about seeing this woman was wearing off. My feet were bouncing up and down, my fingers tapped the sides of the chair.

Where is this woman?

Another thirty minutes passed.

Does she know I'm here? How long are you supposed to wait?

I stared at the clipboard.

Oh, God, I want to knock so badly.

I started going through a deductive reasoning process in my head.

Clearly, she's here. There are other names on the sheet. But did she leave for the day? No. Why would the white noise machine be on? How come no one has come out? Okay, fifteen more minutes and then we're knocking or leaving.

Finally, a woman emerged through the door.

She walked over to me without making eye contact, grabbed the clipboard, and said:

"Leonard?"

I immediately noted that Dr. Baldisseri came across as a crabby, overworked, and angry woman. She looked like Faye Dunaway from *Mommie Dearest*. I felt myself shutting down inside.

How old is this woman? I wondered, as she guided me past the mysterious door and pointed to her couch.

The first words out of her mouth: "What brings you here?"

I perked up and began my dramatic soliloquy of my anxiety, depression, and life story. My heart poured out as my eyes swept the room and saw how empty and small the office was.

She listened for all of five minutes before putting her wrinkled, veiny hand up to stop me and proceeded to ask me a bunch of questions in a much more callous tone.

"I think you've given me enough . . . Any mental health issues in your family?"

"Tons. My mother's crazy."

"And do you have any addiction issues?"

I stopped to think. *I drank a lot in my college days, and I'm having a glass of wine a night these days.*

"Maybe?" I say hesitantly.

She made a note.

Why is she writing? Does she think I'm an alcoholic?

"And are you hearing or seeing things?"

"What do you mean?"

"Is the refrigerator talking to you?" she continued.

"Oh, no."

Crazy, but not that crazy.

Holy shit, what is with all of these random questions? She was rapidly firing through this list, and I barely had time to think about my responses, almost like she was rushing me.

"So what medications are you thinking of taking?"

I froze and paused. I was taken aback because I was looking for someone who would just listen to me talk about my problems. I wasn't ready for medications. My mom was on medications. That wasn't me.

"I was hoping to talk," I said softly.

She sighed and rolled her eyes before bringing her attention back to me with a put-on smile, "Very well, we'll talk."

I didn't realize that psychiatrists were mostly for medication, while psychologists, social workers, and counselors were for talking. Still, Dr. Baldisseri humored me, "listened," and agreed to meet with me weekly for psychotherapy. I felt trapped. It took me so long to get in with her, I figured I might as well give it a try.

From the start, it was clear Dr. Baldisseri was not a listener. I sat in her office week after week regaling her with tales of my failed career, money troubles, and anxiety that I couldn't seem to manage . . .

Wait, is she nodding off, or is she drunk?

During one of our sessions, she was falling asleep or having a stroke or something. Maybe she was just bored by what I was telling her. It became apparent to me that listening wasn't her thing. When she wasn't falling asleep, her general response was a head nod to indicate she agreed with what I said. On the few occasions when she spoke, it was to tell me: "There are pills that can help you manage these feelings."

Two months into treatment, it was obvious that I was not getting better but was merely bringing up a bunch of problems that seemed to have no solutions while all she did was get paid to take a nap. I could have gotten more help talking to a cat cleaning themself than this woman. My anxiety was getting worse every day. My stomach was still in knots, my head always racing with thoughts. I didn't know what to do. It was then when I seriously started to contemplate Dr. Baldisseri's suggestions for medications.

Maybe she's right. Maybe I'm going about this all wrong. Maybe I should try those pills. I mean, I was talking to Nick almost daily about my anxiety. Other people I knew were taking pills and all seemed just fine. Maybe I did need a little chemical help.

I was conflicted about what to do next. My anxious brain struggled to make a decision. I consulted Scott, Nick, and a few close friends about medication. As always, they were little help, because everyone had a different take on it. "No, keep things all natural," some would say. Others would go to the opposite end of the spectrum, "Give it a try, what do you have to lose?"

When you're anxious you want so badly for people to tell you something you haven't thought of or make the decision clearer, but it rarely happens. Even though you know this deep down inside, you keep asking them.

I finally gave in when, one day, Dr. Baldisseri said in her usual callous voice, "You can try them, if you don't like them, you can stop."

This was much like my decision to move to New York the first time. A test. Waiting for my response, she shifted her attention to writing down notes on her paper.

I sat in her office for about ten minutes in silence. I pondered why she put so few things in her office. I wondered if she was married or had a once exciting life. My attention turned to what pills would do to me.

Would they make me feel different? Would it take away my personality? My thoughts fluctuated between, *What if this actually worked?* and *What if this kills me? Maybe she is right. I can always just stop.*

I didn't want to feel this way anymore. Finally, I broke the silence and hesitantly agreed: "Let's try it."

Seemingly relieved that she would not have to be tortured by another one of my anxious tales, she decided to put me on a small dose of Celexa, a very common SSRI antidepressant. Celexa and other Selective Serotonin Reuptake Inhibitors are prescribed to treat depression and anxiety. They're thought to work by increasing serotonin, thus helping to elevate your mood.

Dr. Baldisseri uttered the most words she had ever said to me when she prescribed that pill: "It will take a few weeks for the medicine to work. You shouldn't expect too much from it upfront. If you run into any problems, you can always call me. I'll see you in a month."

What? That's it? That's all we're going to say to each other? It seemed like I had given her the green light to push me out of her office.

"We're not meeting each week?" I asked, baffled that she was putting me on a drug that was about to fuck with my mind but cut back on our sessions.

"No, for medication I can just see you in a month for a follow-up."

I left her office and went directly to the pharmacy to fill my prescription.

That night, I stared at the tiny pill for about an hour—noticing its shape, the numbers imprinted on it. I even licked it to get a sense of its taste. When I was ready, I swallowed the pill with a glass of water and thought, *You can always stop if it doesn't work.* As I climbed into bed, I prayed that this would be the answer to change my life.

The next morning, to my surprise, I felt different. It didn't take weeks for that little pill to kick in, it took hours—and that was a problem. A sadness unlike any other sadness I had ever felt overtook me. All I wanted to do was cry for no apparent reason. If I thought I had experienced sadness before, then this was some next-level shit.

Why can't I stop crying? What did this pill do to me? I tried to figure out what to do next.

Nothing in particular was making me feel sad, but the urge to cry was uncontrollable. I went in and out of crying periods, and when I got to a moment when I wasn't crying and felt I was up to it, I called Dr. Baldisseri, who urged me to stay on the pill for a little longer.

"This is part of the leveling out process," she told me.

I listened to her, but after a couple of days, when I could no longer handle the worsening depression, I quit taking the pill. A few days after that I was back to my usual, moderately depressed self.

As scheduled, I went to my follow-up with Dr. Baldisseri and explained my symptoms to her. I will never forget her exact response, "Perhaps we should try a mood stabilizer next."

Trying to comprehend what she had just said, my body sat there in a frozen state of panic; it was as if she had told me that I only had one month to live.

Remember Anxiety 101? You can't tell an anxious person that the worst is happening to them. I didn't know a lot about these medications, but I knew mood stabilizers were for leveling out a mood, aka, bipolar disorder. This was worse than I expected. In that moment she instilled a fear in me that seemed to validate a very real fear about becoming my mother. I had often suspected my mother had some form of bipolar disorder or something that caused her mood to fluctuate.

Shit, I'm crazier than I had originally suspected.

In her defense, she did explain that I might not be bipolar, but that my body might handle that type of medication better. That moment was it, however. Just like Dr. Pelkington had told me that I might have a tumor, the anxiety-ridden thought that I might be bipolar had been etched in my head and would start devouring me in the upcoming days and months.

She prescribed Trileptal, a common mood stabilizer originally intended to prevent seizures.

When I got home, I ran into Scott's home office and interrupted whatever he was doing, as if I was about to proclaim the worst possible news he would ever hear.

Grabbing him by the shoulders, I ran Dr. Baldisseri's suspicions past Scott, in an attempt to get reassurance that maybe she was wrong.

"Do you think I'm bipolar?" I asked him frantically.

I could see the look of confusion on his face. Scott had no idea how to interpret or answer this question.

"I don't know."

"Do you think I get manic sometimes?" I continued.

He stared at me, and I could tell he was scanning his brain, trying to answer this question as diplomatically as he could. It was as if I had asked him do you think I'm fat, knowing there would be no perfect answer that would suffice.

Hesitantly, he replied, "Well you do get a little intense when you're trying to write."

There it was. Another dagger to the heart. Confirmation from my own partner that I was crazy.

"Do you think I'm like my mother?" I continued, as I started to cry.

"No, are you kidding?" Scott said. He had only met my mother once, but from the little conversation they had that day, and him hearing me talk to her occasionally on the phone, which generally ended up in a screaming match, he knew that I was not like her. Realizing that this was causing me a ton of distress, he gave me a big hug.

Despite his reassurance, I became obsessed and couldn't get the idea of being bipolar out of my head. Everything I read online said that antidepressants may cause a fluctuation of mood in patients with bipolar disorder.

Was Faye Dunaway right? Was my anxiety and energy not that at all, but rather bipolar?

At night I sat up worrying and ruminating about what it would mean if I was bipolar. I feared that I would eventually have a manic episode in which I would lose control of myself. That I would run around the neighborhood naked while the neighbors called the police to take me away. I turned to the Internet, researching everything I could find on the subject; taking every online quiz to help determine if I was bipolar. The results: mixed.

Oh, dear God, is this how it starts?

My research revealed that bipolar was an organic disorder, one that could never leave, only be stabilized.

I'm going to be like my mom, I told myself.

After a couple of days, I took the medication that Dr. Baldisseri prescribed. What better way to test out her theory. It kind of worked and did calm down my anxiety a bit.

Did this mean she was right?

Many questions rattled around in my brain, but whenever I visited Dr. Baldisseri she had no patience to answer them. My head was exploding with thoughts that I couldn't process, and when it became too much, I decided it was time to go back to my gut reaction and find a person to talk to, someone who would listen.

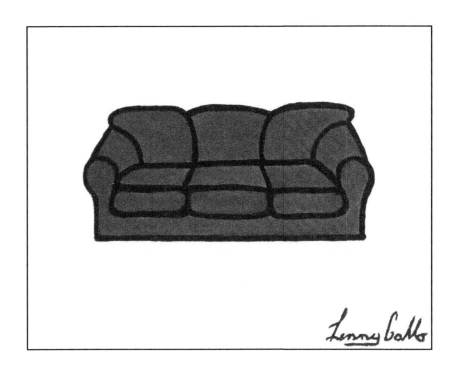

Talk Therapy: A Tribute, 2012, oil on canvas, 12" x 16".

CHAPTER 6
The Comfy Couch

Another lengthy search began, this time to find a therapist. Much like the psychiatrists, many of my top choices were not seeing new patients. Some of them never even returned my phone calls. Message after message was left until, finally, I got a return call from a woman who agreed to see me for an intake.

I liked Dr. Zabel from the start. Her office was warm and friendly. She had a plush couch, and positive affirmations and trinkets were spread all over.

Dr. Zabel was a psychologist and said, "A lot of psychiatrists these days don't always have the time to do traditional talk therapy."

Don't have time? Why the fuck do they make so much money if they don't have time.

She recommended that Dr. Baldisseri be strictly for medication, while she and I would talk about whatever I would like.

"What would you like to talk about?" she asked as she leaned closer to me.

I paused for a moment and looked her in the eyes, trying to assess if I could open up to this woman. Did she already have an opinion formed of me?

My hands were clenching the sides of the comfy couch. Hesitantly, I told her, "I'm worried I might be bipolar."

In her calming voice she said, "Okay, let's figure that out then."

I let out more: "And my acting career sucks."

"We can talk about that too."

My hands still gripped the couch, as if that action would save me as I worked up the courage to say the thing that scared me the most: "And I'm worried about my relationship with my partner."

Without a pause she said, "A lot of people have that concern."

Nothing was off the table. Dr. Zabel made me feel that I could engage with her. She was empathetic and caring. She was on time.

Thank God, finally someone who would listen to my anxious ass.

I always felt optimistic when I left her office. As we delved deeper into my problems, I started to look forward to our weekly sessions and would get upset when our time was up. This was the one space where I could say anything and not feel judged. She helped me work through much of my anxiety and depression. But Dr. Baldisseri's words haunted me, maybe what was going on in my brain was unfixable.

In addition to talking to Dr. Zabel, I worked with Dr. Baldisseri to keep trying pills. The Trileptal wasn't working that well. It made me slightly less anxious but didn't do much for the racing thoughts.

"Perhaps we need to add something along with this medicine," Dr. Baldisseri said during one of our visits.

Great. Let's try and solve this problem, I thought. If I was bipolar, at the very least I wanted it managed before it became worse.

We went through a series of trial and error with more types of medication: Wellbutrin, Buspar, Zoloft, and Paxil, all with no success.

I should point out that some of these medicines did help with my anxiety and depression, but they came with awful side effects—everything from weight gain to . . .

Shit, why can't I get my dick hard? The label warned of possible erectile dysfunction. I verified this one day as I tried to jerk off in the bathroom. After forty-five minutes of rubbing myself raw, I gave up.

When I found a pill that made me feel better, I got upset because it would cause all these other problems. Not many men in their late twenties would be willing to accept erectile dysfunction as an acceptable tradeoff for happiness.

During this whole time of trying pills, I started to see the benefits of talk therapy. Working with Dr. Zabel, I was able to figure out some stuff in my life. One of the big issues we were dealing with was working through the fears I had about my future and my current career.

I still wanted to continue with my acting, but I realized that my reasons for wanting to do so were more about connecting with others and self-expression versus the reality of what the business was. It was still something I wanted to pursue, but I wanted it to be more on my terms. And I wanted to feel good about the parts I was taking, not trying to base my living on it.

My hands and wrists hurt from being a massage therapist, and I knew that even with the best body mechanics, massage therapy would have a cap on it. Graduate school was always something I saw in my future; I just wasn't always sure for what.

"Why not look at everything?" Dr. Zabel suggested during one of our appointments.

Why the hell not? I thought.

With the help of Dr. Zabel, I spent all of 2010 researching programs that might interest me. Everything was on the table: graphic designer, a doctorate in theatre history, counseling, social work, psychology, marine biology, and nursing. I searched the Internet, visited schools, attended workshops and open houses, and talked to individuals in these fields. It felt good to work toward something again. My anxious brain wanted to be absolutely sure that I would enjoy the education I was about to spend tens of thousands of dollars on, money that I didn't have. I was still paying off loans from my undergraduate degree in theatre.

After tons of research and contemplation, I settled on counseling. It felt like a natural transition from the work I had done as a massage therapist and actor, and I liked how it afforded me the possibility of one day having my own private practice and being on the other side of the couch. I could do my acting, art, and writing on my terms. Talking to people also came naturally and I loved listening to them. Most of the time when I massaged people, I felt like I already was a talk therapist. My massages were good, but clients came to me to talk, to share their lives with me, and I really took in their stories.

I'd be lying if I didn't admit that counseling fascinated me partly because I wanted to understand myself better. People also intrigued me, and I wanted to understand how their past influenced their present and how all this talking helped.

After a chance encounter at a Starbucks with a longtime massage client, I changed my mind and decided that social work would be a better choice for me. He explained the different licensing requirements between counseling and social work and how that might impact my career prospects.

Social Work had been around a lot longer than counseling, which was still an evolving field. Even though the two degrees were virtually the same, with a few minor differences in the curriculum, social work was a straightforward path.

Considering what I had been through with my massage licenses, and not wanting to make the same mistake, I did my research and compared the licensing requirements of counseling versus social work in New Jersey and other possible states that I would even remotely consider living in. Social Work requirements were mostly standardized, while counseling was vastly different. Social Work it was.

I felt incredibly sad to give up trying to make a living as a professional actor. Even if I wasn't getting the best parts or making it as far as I hoped, it was still exciting to be an actor. Whenever I would get into this state of mind, Dr. Zabel would reframe me.

"You're still going to be able to act, but now you don't have to take every part that comes your way. You can be more selective, and, as you said, do it on your terms," she would say.

"But how am I going to express myself as a therapist?"

"What the hell do you think I've been doing with you?" she said, half-jokingly, half-serious. "Your life experiences and proper training will allow you to guide other people. You said it yourself, there's a difference between the business of acting versus the art of acting."

I was hopeful that my new path would give me the flexibility to go back and pursue my art and acting, the way I wanted—just not as a starving artist.

In 2011, I applied to tons of graduate schools in social work and got into every one except for the University of Pennsylvania. "You wrote one of the best admissions essays I've ever seen, but you just don't have a strong enough background in psychology. Take a class in psychology and reapply next year," said the admissions officer who interviewed me.

Girl! I'm an actor who lived with a psychopath for a mother, and I practically mediated my parents' divorce. If that isn't sufficient psychology for you, then your Ivy League pretentious self can kiss my ass. Sorry, Dad, no Ivy Leaguers are coming out of this generation.

"I'll think about it," I told her.

With the University of Pennsylvania out of the way, the decision boiled down to three schools: New York University, Loyola University in Chicago, and Fordham in New York. I couldn't believe that I, of all people, got into these schools!

Dr. Zabel and I were also tackling my relationship with Scott and the resentment I felt.

"You need to talk to him, tell him how you're feeling," she said frequently in our sessions.

This felt so difficult. "How can I do that?" I asked. "Talking to him feels like it would be confronting him, and that's not who I am."

One reason I applied to Loyola in Chicago was that I knew things were coming to a head with Scott. Well, at least coming to a head in my mind, but I learned in therapy that I wasn't going to be able to hold my feelings in forever. I wanted an out in case Scott and I couldn't resolve some of what we were going through. But I would have to tell Scott exactly what the problems were, since he was unaware of all the unspoken thoughts in my brain.

I don't know what came over me one day when I left Dr. Zabel's office. Maybe it was the pressure of having to decide what school to go to; maybe I had gained some courage; maybe I had just had enough. I felt a heaviness in my chest and a surge of energy that could not be tamed. It was so intense that, as that surge jolted through my brain, I thought I would pass out. My buried and suppressed feelings about our relationship couldn't be held in anymore. No part of my body would let me hold them in, and the words tumbled out of my mouth as I walked into Scott's office.

I felt lightheaded and on the verge of having a panic attack, because I knew that what I was about to do was going to change the course of both of our lives.

Scott was sitting at his computer. In a serious tone, I said, "We need to talk."

Tears dropped down my face as my feelings came pouring out.

Scott sat motionless and looked worried and concerned by just the sight of me.

"What's wrong?" he said.

I went through a prewritten list of everything that I believed was wrong in our relationship: how I disliked cooking dinner every night and how I never got to pick the restaurant when we went out. I repeated my discontent that he used a towel only once. I told him I resented not being able to go on a tour and expressed my hatred that he had moved us to the suburbs.

It took every ounce of courage I had to tell Scott, "I feel like you took my independence, and I don't feel as though I had a say in this relationship."

He seemed shocked at what was being thrown at him, but I knew I needed the freedom to pursue my life on my terms and not feel guilted into being held back. Sobbing profusely, I said what would be the hardest thing I would ever tell him, "I'm not sure I love you anymore." The more I spoke, the more the weight on my chest lifted.

Scott's eyes watered, and he let a few tears roll down his cheeks.

There was a long pause.

"I don't know how to respond," he said. "I don't know how to fix this."

My diatribe had come to an end. I covered my face as if to hide behind a shield. Weeping, choking on my words, I whispered, "I don't know if we can."

That night as we lay in bed, I heard Scott crying himself to sleep but trying to hide it from me. I turned around and put my arm around him, unsure of what to do about this disaster I had just unleashed on our household. He turned toward me, and like a child might grab their blanket, he held me and began to sob. "I love you. I don't want you to leave," he said.

All I could do was hold him as I had no words left in me. And all I could think was: *What happens now?*

I wasn't sure what I really wanted from him. I wasn't sure what I wanted him to say or do. Getting my feelings out lifted a weight from me, but now I would have to deal with the repercussions, and a new weight of worry would take its place.

What happens now?

That next week we had moments of discussion combined with fighting. Until this point, we never really fought. Let me revise that statement: I never really fought. It felt empowering, because I wasn't keeping my emotions inside anymore. I learned from Dr. Zabel how to express myself in a healthy way.

Our fights soon turned into problem solving, with Scott and me both offering suggestions. We sat on our couch one day, and he apologized for buying the house without consulting me first and said that he would be open to a possible move someday when finances were different, if I was still unhappy out here.

"I'm sorry I didn't appreciate your effort with the cooking and cleaning," he continued. It felt good to be acknowledged, but taking my share of responsibility, too, I responded, "That was stupid for me to say. I like cooking, just not every night, but I do want a say when we eat out."

The most important thing Scott told me was that going forward he wouldn't hold me back from anything I wanted to do. I apologized for unleashing my anxious wrath on him. He looked at me with his hurt brown eyes and asked if we could give it another try. "Can we see what happens?"

I wasn't sure. I felt so confused. And I was upset with myself for causing another human being that kind of anguish. What was the right next step? How were we going to repair all of this?

"I want you to go to Fordham; I know that's where you want to go," he said. He was right, it was my top choice, but I would never feel right about going there if we couldn't come to a resolution about us.

"Seeing what happens" didn't provide the certainty my brain craved. It wasn't the perfect fix, but did I really want to throw away our relationship, especially since he was acknowledging his insensitivity and wanted to try?

"I love you so much," he told me. I said it back, but I wasn't sure it was entirely true.

After taking time to think it over, I agreed to give it a try—a final try. But how this would play out would be anybody's guess. Looking back, I don't think I wanted to lose or leave Scott. What I wanted was to feel like an equal in our relationship. We held each other, our pending future looming in the distance. Balance was restored for the moment.

"How do you feel about working through things and seeing where it goes?" Dr. Zabel asked at our next session.

"It's not a perfect solution, but I think I can live with it for now," I told her.

She smiled at me proudly, glad that I expressed my feelings to Scott and pleased to hear that I was being flexible. "I guess that narrows your school decision," she said.

I had definitely narrowed down the schools. I could go to either NYU or Fordham, but according to the *Newsweek* reports on top schools for social work, Fordham came ahead of NYU. Also, NYU felt very pretentious. Instinctually, Fordham felt right for me.

The day I made the decision to go to Fordham, I stared out of our front window and wondered what this new future would bring. I saw two doves sitting on a tree branch, making a shit-ton of noise.

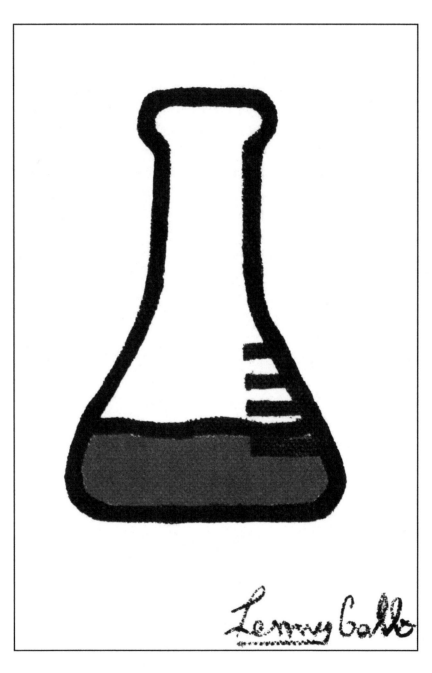

Chemistry Experiment, 2012, oil on canvas, 4" x 6".

CHAPTER 7
Antipsychotics

Despite the progress I made in therapy, from getting into graduate school and working through relationship issues, I still couldn't manage this fucking anxiety. And there was one big question we had not gotten the answer to . . .

"What if I have a manic episode at Fordham?" I said to Dr. Zabel during one of our sessions.

The seed of me needing a mood stabilizer that Dr. Baldisseri had planted was starting to sprout.

With a sigh and a look that had an undertone that implied, "We've had this conversation before," Dr. Zabel responded. "Lenny, I really don't think you're bipolar."

"How do you know that?"

I wanted to believe her, but I could not get that possibility out of my head. And why did she say, "really don't think." She didn't know for sure. What if she was wrong?

"You're not showing signs of this. I work with people who are bipolar, and that doesn't fit you."

Practically before the words were out of her mouth I rebutted, "Then why did that first pill I took cause changes in my mood?"

"Some people have bad side effects from medications."

That answer wasn't good enough for me. Dr. Zabel never believed I was bipolar and always thought this was anxiety and depression. She thought I might have to accept the level of comfort I was getting with Trileptal, which was the only pill I could handle.

Even if she was right and that was the case, I didn't want Dr. Baldisseri to be a fixture in my life anymore. I had enough of her inability to connect with me on a human level. Dr. Zabel and I agreed that if I didn't get along with Dr. Baldisseri, I could find a new psychiatrist.

Looking back, I think Dr. Zabel hoped that a different psychiatrist might be able to help put the bipolar debate to rest and give me a different perspective. I went through another lengthy search and wait time to find my new psychiatrist.

What is with these psychiatrists' offices?

I sat in the waiting room of another psychiatrist, whose office didn't seem to be much better than Dr. Baldisseri's. His was more sterile and hospital-like than hers, and it, too, felt cold and uninviting.

During the initial intake, Dr. Pavlichuk seemed slightly more capable of listening than his predecessor. He was an older man with a private office in Passaic. He listened to my background, and rather than try to debate the bipolar suspicion, he told me, "We need to investigate a different class of medication."

I hadn't even thought about this. Tell me more . . .

I was curious. I thought I was fully versed in all the mental health medications, but was there something I hadn't heard of?

With assuredness he explained, "These pills work for everything; it's just a dosing issue. For anxiety, lower doses are used, schizophrenia, slightly higher. They can treat a multitude of different mental health issues, and there are very few reports of sexual side effects."

Hmm . . . Something that will treat whatever is going on with me and I'll be able to have sex? Impressive.

What he was referring to was a class of medications known as antipsy-chotics. At this time there was a big push from drug companies for this class of medication. They were marketing these drugs to everyday consumers. You've probably seen the commercials:

"Is your antidepressant not enough?" and "Are you still having those rough days on your antidepressant? Talk to your doctor about . . ." the announcer said in a soft, calming tone.

These pills sounded like a miracle, and the research carried out by the pharmaceutical companies was quite convincing.

Hesitant but also excited, I asked: "So, you can take these for anything?"

"Yep. It's just about dosing," he answered in a pleasant tone.

"And what *are* the side effects?" I asked, wanting to do my due diligence. It was nice that I would be able to have sex, but what else could happen?

He started writing on his prescription pad and said, "People usually tolerate them very well."

I paused, not sure what to think, because he hadn't answered my question, but I was still open to the idea. I could research side effects when I got home.

"And how long do they take to work?"

"Usually pretty quickly, within a few days."

Wow. Why wasn't everyone on these?

These pills did seem impressive. I decided to try one: Abilify.

I'll never forget the first day of that pill. As I did with all the new medications I ever took, I popped the pill at night in case it made me nauseous. When I woke up in the morning I felt like a new person. My mood was up, and I had a good energy. The thoughts that had been invading my brain weren't there. I actually remember feeling happy. Was this a placebo effect? It didn't matter. I was ready to conquer the world.

This shit is awesome, I told myself. *Did we just find the answer?*

I decided that I wanted to work with Dr. Pavlichuk, so I called Dr. Baldisseri to cancel my follow-up appointment. She didn't care. Why would she? People were so desperate to use their insurance for their mental health, she would fill my space quickly.

Things were good for the first couple of days, and I thought I was going to be done with this nightmare. On day three, however, something strange happened. Scott and I were in the city, checking out a new show on Broadway. My body started to shake with that antsy feeling.

By the time we went to dinner, it was getting worse. I went from calm and blissful to what seemed like a panic attack and could barely get through the meal. Scott encouraged me to do some breathing exercises as we went through the Lincoln Tunnel on our drive home. When we walked in the door, I was sweating, and my heart was racing. All I wanted to do was crawl in bed. This did not feel right. I was upset, because I really wanted this to be the answer, but it seemed like my body was too sensitive for this stuff. Having ruined our night out, I decided it was finally time to call it quits with medicine.

I phoned Dr. Pavlichuk the next day and told him what was happening. He told me to stop the pill and we could discuss it at our next appointment.

I was getting sick of all these pills. Was Dr. Zabel right? Would I have to just stick with the minimal benefits from the one pill that gave me a little relief and call it a day?

"We probably found the right class of medicine for you, since you felt good at first. Now we just need to find one that doesn't cause these symptoms," said Doctor Pavlichuk at our next visit. That reassured me somewhat, but every time I went on one of these pills I got unbearable side effects, and when they did work, they didn't work that well.

"I think there might be a better one for you," Dr. Pavlichuk said, trying to encourage me that all was not lost with medication and that there still might be hope.

Very hesitantly I told him, "I don't know if want to stick with medication anymore. Maybe I just stay with the Trileptal."

"That's fine. There is this newer one that's similar. It should be covered by your insurance, and it doesn't have much in the way of reported side effects. It might be better for you if you want to give that one a try. A lot of people report shakiness on Abilify."

I wanted so much to believe that he was right, even though a nagging voice in my head told me to stay away. But I hardly ever listened to that little fucker in my head and kiboshed its attempts to try and stop me.

After a few moments of contemplation, I gave the green light for this final pill. "Okay. Let's give it a go, but this is it."

Baffled and furious, Dr. Zabel threw her hands up in the air as I sat in her office for our weekly visit. "Why is he putting you on antipsychotics?"

Dr. Zabel seemed alarmed that we were going down this route, and we spent most of the session talking about it.

"He thinks we're in the right class of medication," I told her.

"I think I should call him. This is heavy-duty stuff you're on. They're also dangerous. This is what they put people with schizophrenia on."

Realizing what she had just said, she looked at me and saw the look of horror on my face.

"You don't have schizophrenia."

She knew me well enough to know that she had to watch what to say around me. She took Anxiety 101.

I was open to her calling him, but part of me wanted to believe Dr. Pavlichuk. Those first few days on Abilify I really did feel like a new person. Nothing bothered me.

"You can call him, but I think after this I want to put medicines on hold and just stick with the Trileptal and talking. Maybe doing more yoga. I'm sick of trying these things, but if this one works . . . I don't know. This will be the last one I try."

She held back what she probably really wanted to say and said, "You're done after this?"

"I'm done."

Famous last words.

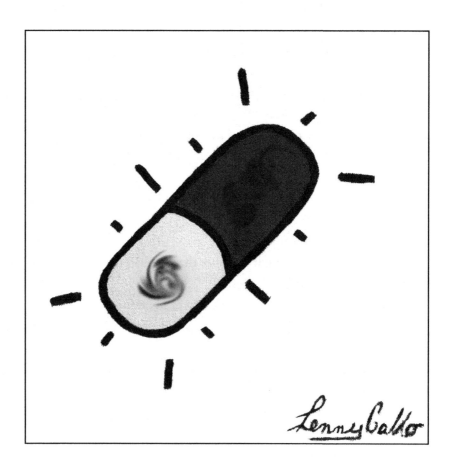

Title Censored One, 2012, oil on canvas, 12" x 12".

CHAPTER 8
"That Was It!"

Geodon was the drug of choice for this final round. Like many of the other pills I had taken, this one started out fine.

Scott and I were coming home one night. We were trying to spend as much time together as we could, because we knew that once I started grad school I wouldn't have all this free time. We were also trying to rebuild our relationship and connect more: talking a lot more and really listening to each other. As we were getting ready for bed, I noticed my heart racing.

"Something doesn't feel right," I said as I lay next to him, trying not to panic.

"What's wrong?" he asked, half asleep.

I grabbed his hand and placed it on my chest. "My heart is racing. Feel."

My heart wasn't just racing. Putting my middle and index fingers on the carotid artery in my neck, I was able to measure the resting beats per minute.

"It's one-forty," I told Scott. (I knew that a normal resting heartbeat was sixty to one hundred beats per minute.)

"It does feel a little fast. Try and breathe," he said, concerned but practically asleep. "Do you need anything?"

"I think I'll be fine. I think I'm going to try and sleep this off."

Scott turned to hug me and said, "I'm here if you need anything."

In that moment I thought about all the medicine I had taken up until now and how Dr. Zabel was right.

I didn't like this feeling in my chest. I didn't like what these things were doing to me.

"*Fuck this!!!* I'm done. I'm done with these things!" I proclaimed emphatically.

Scott seemed relieved: "Good, you can do this naturally. I'm sick of these pills ruining your days." Even though he didn't like me putting these pills in my body, Scott always tried to be supportive through this process.

That was it. I was done with pharmaceuticals. This shit was way too complicated, and I had tried enough.

The following morning I called Dr. Pavlichuk and left a voice message saying that I wanted to discontinue *all* medication and stick with things the natural way. I felt great leaving him that message. Medication wasn't something for me. I'd be lying if I said that the thought of being bipolar didn't scare me, but if I was, it didn't seem like there was going to be a medication that would help me manage it. I would just have to manage the way I always had. And now that I had a therapist, I felt more confident working through my problems as opposed to avoiding them.

Dr. Pavlichuk returned my call later that afternoon: "That's fine. You can just stop taking the meds. You haven't been on them that long. Let's just schedule a follow-up in two weeks to make sure everything is okay."

Sounded good to me. I was free. As I ended the phone conversation, I felt a sense of mental clarity and freedom. Physically, however, my body was still feeling some of the effects of getting the medicine out of my system.

About a week after being off the pills, I noticed that my heart was still going through periods where it was racing, and my energy was increasingly intense. That Saturday, my friend Nick and I were going to see a movie. It was his treat to celebrate my decision to go to Fordham.

"Are you excited for the fall?" he asked as he drove us to the movie theater.

I thought about how far I had come, then I said, "You know what, I am."

As he proceeded down the streets of New Jersey he continued, "You should be. And what are you doing about the pills?"

"I'm done. That last one made my heart race. I thought I was going to have to go to the hospital. It still races, but not as bad as it had been."

An unsettling question ran through my mind, *Why was it taking so long for this pill to work its way through me*? But I pushed this aside, wanting to enjoy the night.

"Give it a couple of days, let it work out of your system," Nick said.

In the theatre we sat in the new, reclining seats of this renovated cinema. You could order food and have it brought to your seats—very fancy and chic. I ordered a burger, and Nick ordered a salad. He claimed he was not cheating on his diet, yet his hand casually managed to make its way over to my basket of fries. The smell of movie theatre popcorn filled the auditorium, and I sat back in my seat, trying to be present for this moment. Even though my body was still working out the medication, I had an inner glow from being with my friend. We watched the movie, and afterward we talked in anticipation of our futures. The night ended early, because I had to work in the morning.

As I walked in the door that night, I saw Scott sitting on the couch watching *The Daily Show with Jon Stewart*.

"How was the movie?" he asked.

"It was okay," I said. "I have to stop letting Nick pick the movies."

"Okay, honey. Don't forget we have Tiff, Mike, and Justin coming tomorrow."

"Great." But after a moment, I thought about what tomorrow was. There was a very important event happening the next night, and I didn't want my plans derailed by us having houseguests.

"Wait … we're still watching the series finale of *Desperate House-wives* and having pizza, right?"

"Yes, I told them. Tiff watches it, too, and wants to see it."

"When I get off work on Sunday, I want to shower, eat pizza, gorge, and do nothing but watch the finale," I responded.

Scott smiled at me and turned his attention to my body. "How are you feeling?"

"My heart is still racing, but not as bad. I think I want to go for a quick walk before I go to bed and get some of this energy out."

I strolled up and down the side streets in Verona taking in the night air; my head tilted toward the sky. Everything, other than my body, felt so right. My heart was still racing from the Geodon working out of my system, but I didn't care. I didn't feel empty anymore, and I had some direction in my life again. I thought about how far I had made it and the fun I was having that year, 2012, which was also when I turned thirty. In January, some friends from Chicago came to visit; we had a blast celebrating in New York City.

And, on that night in May, my face beamed as I looked up at the sky and thought about my next steps; *I can't believe you got in and are going to Fordham.* Life for me was about to change. I finally felt like I was getting closer to me again.

The next morning was Mother's Day, which was always a difficult day for me because of my relationship with my mother. But it didn't matter. I was ready for this new path.

But I wish I knew then what I know now. I wish I had fully absorbed and appreciated all aspects of that night. I wish I could go back to those moments, because it was the last time I would ever feel a sense of naiveté and optimism about my future. It would be the last night I would ever feel like my old self. Edmund had been working in the background that week, and he was ready to start showing himself.

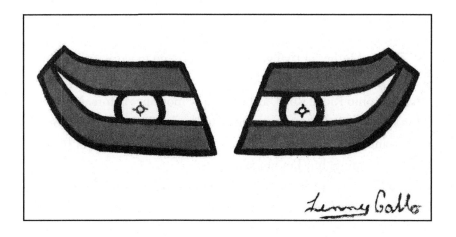

Taillights, 2012, oil on canvas, 9" x 12".

CHAPTER 9
Taillights

On Mother's Day I got into my car to go to work, still feeling a little uneasy. I was taking my usual route and made a right turn onto Ridge Road, as I had many mornings before. Normally, I don't pay much attention to other cars on the road other than for the usual standard safety stuff. I think it was a black Mercedes in front of me that morning, but I'm not sure.

I didn't know what was happening in my brain, but I soon became fixated on the taillights of that car. I wasn't just fixated. I felt extremely panicked by them and had this sense of terror. The taillights were bright red. It felt like they were glaring at me. They projected an ominous presence of evil, almost as if they were a doorway to hell and the eyes of Satan himself saying: "I'm coming for you." Suddenly I snapped out of it.

What the fuck was that? I wondered.

I didn't know what to make of the phenomenon that I had just experienced. I focused my eyes back on the road and came back to reality. But, before I could reflect on what had just happened, the terror set in again. This terror was unlike anything I'd experienced before. No part of me could comprehend what was going on, but the fear permeating my body made me shake in horror. I tried to reason with it: "Okay, this is crazy, snap out of it," but as soon as I had a clear thought, the terror came back, and it would come back again, and again, and again.

Ridge Road is long, and it seemed that the Mercedes was going to be traveling the entire length of it with me.

Eventually, I made it to the parking lot. In my moments of sanity, I assumed this was the medication working out of my body. I tried not to give it much thought, but this thing was relentless. The sense of terror wouldn't leave me. As I approached the entrance to work and walked in, I became paranoid and believed that people were staring at me and knew what was going on inside my head. The image of those taillights persisted.

"Hey, Lenny? How are you?" one of the receptionists said.

I didn't know how to answer that simple question, which that day seemed very complex. I tried to sound as normal and sane as I possibly could, choosing my words very carefully. "I'm doing good," I said very slowly, with my teeth clenched and a fake smile adorning my face, trying not to evoke any suspicion from her or the others who started coming near me.

I walked directly to the breakroom, where I put down my things and kept the conversation light with everyone. My heart was racing, my breathing was getting faster. I avoided eye contact with my coworkers and made my way into the massage room where I would be working for the day.

Once there I did some deep breathing to calm myself down, but that wasn't working. Nothing I tried helped. *What the fuck is happening to me?*

This was going to be a rough day. One of the most popular gifts to get Mom on Mother's Day is a massage, and we were booked in advance for weeks. I had seven clients back-to-back to massage in that dark room with nothing but my paranoid thoughts. No one would be canceling today.

"My husband won't let me get the bathroom renovated until next year," said one client as I worked on her callused feet.

Shut up, you entitled shit! Who gives a fuck about your Goddamn bathroom? Clearly, I'm having a breakdown. Why am I so scared? Why am I still thinking about those taillights? What am I actually scared of? Calm down . . . Just try and calm down.

"Oh, no, that's awful," I responded.

Everything made me anxious and paranoid that day, and I couldn't stop my head from going in and out of this terror.

During one session, when the client was face down on the table, I started to cry. *Again?* I thought. *What is happening to me? Am I seriously going crazy?*

A tear fell from my eye and landed on her back.

Oh, God, did she feel that? As I bent down to check, I heard her snoring. *Let's just rub that in with some cream.*

The intensity of this thing felt as if it would explode inside me. Throughout the day, to try and stay as sane as I possibly could, I focused my attention on each part of the body as I massaged my clients, and like a Gregorian chant, I kept repeating:

Five more minutes on the calf,
two more minutes on the calf,
one more leg, then to the feet.
You've got this. Finish the feet, get them water, clean your room.

When the day finally came to an end, I ran past the front desk without collecting my tips, got in my car, and drove home, making a conscious effort not to stare at any taillights. I tried to make sense of this in my moments of clarity, but the anxiety and pure terror I was feeling couldn't be compared to anything I had ever felt before.

Just focus on something else and try to distract yourself. The only other thing I could think of was how I should probably call my mother as a courtesy and wish her a happy Mother's Day. I didn't want to call her. My relationship with my mother was becoming more and more complicated and had reached the point where the slightest thing I said would create a fight. If I didn't call her, however, I knew she would use this against me at some point. Assessing the state I was in, I figured it was best that I cut my losses this holiday and take her screaming at me some other time.

Once back home, I wanted to tell Scott what was happening to me. Our houseguests had arrived, and their younger son was incredibly rambunctious, running around our house.

Fucking children. This is so not the time for this.

"Hi, Lenny, how've you been?" said Tiff.

Fuck I've got to make small talk.

"Good. Justin's getting so big," I said with a smile, trying to keep up the appearance that I was completely normal and sane.

Noticing that I was clearly not myself, Scott pulled me aside in our bedroom.

"Are you going to be okay for pizza and *Desperate Housewives*?"

I think I might be possessed by the time the night is over, but let's talk about pizza and TV right now.

"Yeah. I just need to sit on the couch and relax."

And throw this child out a window.

I had Mondays off, so I decided that tomorrow would be a day to relax and let the final bits of this medication work out of me.

I couldn't tell you much about the *Desperate Housewives'* series finale. I was so paralyzed by fear, it took all my effort to keep it together in front of our houseguests so as not to alarm them. I was trapped in my head. Everything was frightening me: loud noises from the TV, the sound of our guest's child running around the house.

Maybe I just needed to sleep this off, I thought, as if this were some sort of hangover.

After putting up with as much of other people as I could for one day, I decided to try and sleep. I told Scott and our guests that I was going to go to bed early that night. I vowed to myself that if this didn't get better by morning, I would get Pavlichuk on the phone.

All that night I sat in bed trying to force myself to sleep, doing as much deep breathing as I could to keep my nerves calm, but nothing seemed to be working.

Oh, Edmund. I still recall those first moments with you. In a million years I could never have anticipated your next steps.

I managed to get a few hours of sleep, but the next morning I was worse than the day before. The terror continued to advance, retreat, and advance again. I don't know what I was supposed to be frightened of, but the feeling that something was going to harm me kept invading my brain. And, I had a new symptom: I could not sit still. When I tried, I would rock back and forth, much like you see psychiatric patients do in a movie. I felt like I was crawling out of my skin. Edmund was physically taking over my body.

As soon as the clock hit 9:00 a.m., the moment when the doctor's answering service switched off and the office answered calls, I phoned Dr. Pavlichuk. Emblazoned in my mind were his first words, "Shit, we may have opened a Pandora's box that we might not be able to shut. You should come in right away."

Oh, God. Pandora's box!

I told him, "Okay," not knowing what else to say, but my hopes for a quick resolution to whatever was happening to me faded with his comment. I wailed hysterically and called for Scott. "I can't sit still. I can't sit still. He wants to see me as soon as I can get there."

This was all so crazy and surreal. What was happening to me? I called Dr. Zabel to tell her what was going on.

Not sure of how to respond, she tried her best to calm me down. "You're probably just having a bad reaction to the medicine. Let's see what happens after you see the psychiatrist. Please keep me in the loop."

Dr. Zabel tried desperately to reassure me that I would be okay, but by now I was inconsolable.

I didn't feel comfortable driving, so I went with Scott to see Dr. Pavlichuk. This was the first time Scott had been involved fully in the whole process of my mental healthcare. I also didn't feel able to hear or absorb everything that would be talked about at that meeting, so I wanted him there. Out of naiveté, I don't think Scott ever thought to question any of what I was doing with these doctors. He trusted my judgment on these things. In moments of crisis, however, the one thing I could always count on Scott for was to dive into action.

We walked into Dr. Pavlichuk's office and waited for him to come get us. Scott tried to console me. "We're going to get you better," he said calmly, as if this were a cut that needed stitches.

I was in a different world altogether, lost in my head, trying to keep myself from going crazy. The only thing I remember Dr. Pavlichuk saying was that he was shutting down his practice.

He wrote a prescription for 120 tablets of .5 milligrams of Ativan, a benzodiazepine. He told me to take them as needed until I felt better and that I would need to find a new psychiatrist to help manage these new symptoms.

"You're leaving?" was the only thing I could get out of my mouth. I wanted to scream at this man, but all I was able to do was sit in disbelief, coming in and out of my paranoid thoughts. Now that I was having some sort of mental health crisis, the one person I depended on to help me was leaving.

I may not have been able to yell at this man, but Scott had no trouble finding the words that wouldn't come to me. The two of them got into a screaming match. The word "fuck" coming from Scott, and "You're being belligerent," coming from Dr. Pavlichuk were about the only things I could make out.

The next thing I remember was being back in Scott's car. Much like he did when he was in traffic, Scott shouted, "That man is a quack."

Briefly, I came back to reality. As Scott drove, I could tell he was very anxious. When he got anxious, he became very quiet, and his eyes shifted all over the place. In a weird way, I remember being calmed by his frustration and anxiety. It was as if for a few moments he absorbed my anxiety, giving me a chance to breathe.

"What do I do?" I said softly to him.

In as calm a voice as he could muster, Scott looked at me, taking his eyes off the road for a minute. "I don't know, but we'll figure this out."

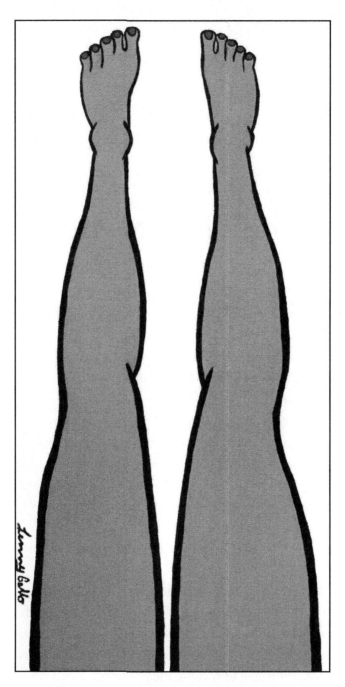

Legs, 2012, oil on canvas, 10" x 20".

CHAPTER 10
The Light Switch

D r. Zabel suggested that I try the Ativan to see if it helped calm my brain a bit. Even though medicine wasn't her scope of practice, she knew that this was not the usual me. I called my boss and took a few sick days. There was no way I was working again in this condition.

The next couple of days I sat on the floor in a corner of our living room, unable to stop rocking back and forth, holding my legs and feet in an attempt to keep them from moving, rubbing my shoulders in my efforts to self-soothe this thing.

At night, sleep for both Scott and me was very hard as I came in and out of these bits of terror.

"Scott, the light switch," I said as he was trying to fall asleep.

"What?"

"It's staring at me," I said horrified.

Our light switch had an orange dot that glowed at night. It alarmed me and brought me back to that day in the car with the taillights.

"There's nothing wrong with the light switch," he said, chuckling from anxiety, yet trying to reassure me.

"No, it feels like it's staring at me."

I thought back to something Dr. Baldisseri had asked me when I was seeing her at that moment, and trying to keep something so terrifying a little lighter, I told Scott, "Hey, maybe the refrigerator will start talking to me next."

We both laughed in an uncomfortable way, in disbelief at what was happening. Neither of us knew how to act or think. Never completely did I lose touch with reality, but felt I was on the verge and that at any moment the pendulum would swing too far in one direction, and I would no longer be in control of my body or mind. I took the Ativan as needed up to four times a day, but when that didn't seem to be working, and when it became too much to bear, I told Scott he needed to take me to the ER.

"Lenny, maybe you should wait this out," said Dr. Zabel when I called to let her know what was happening. "I'm afraid if you go to the ER, they're going to make whatever this is worse."

"I don't know if I can." I thought about what she said, but this thing felt so much bigger than me. How could I just wait this out? This thing inside of me kept me terrified and moving all day and night. Someone needed to tell me what I was dealing with and what was going on.

But You're Functioning, 2012, oil on canvas, 11" x 14".

CHAPTER 11
"But You're Functioning."

Later that night we went to Memorial Hospital's ER. People packed the waiting room with issues from broken bones to the elderly, who were being carted in on stretchers and appeared to be taking their final breaths of life. The place was incredibly chaotic. There were so many people, even after I was admitted Scott and I had to sit on a bed in the hallway. We were there for many hours, me rocking back and forth, Scott rubbing my back. I could taste the sterile smell of disinfectant and bleach. A woman came around with sandwiches and juice boxes. I couldn't eat, but Scott had a sandwich.

"This tastes awful," Scott said, talking with his mouth full.

I smiled. As much as I would have loved to critique the food with him that night, I was lost in my thoughts of what was wrong with me. Despite all the chaos, I believed that I was in the best place for me and that someone would eventually come to tell me what was going on.

Finally, a doctor came and started to ask generic questions about my overall health.

"Do you smoke? How is your blood pressure?" he asked quickly, trying to assess in between patients.

He listened to my heart and palpated the lymph nodes of my neck, which felt incredibly ridiculous, as if these simple tests could reveal anything relevant to my immediate problem. When he asked me what was going on, I barely got a few words out before he stopped me by saying, "Someone from mental health will be here shortly."

We waited again. Soon a young, blonde woman approached. She was a social worker. Great, this is what I was going to be when I graduated. Let's see her in action.

"How are you doing?" she said in that voice you use when you're talking to a child.

"Not good," I said, trying to keep myself from squirming off the bed.

"What's going on?"

"I'm not sure. I stopped taking this medication that a psychiatrist prescribed for me and I started getting terrifying thoughts, and now I can't stop moving. I was only on the meds for a few days." I paused for a moment from my nonstop narrative and said, "I didn't have any of these problems prior to this. This only started once I got off the meds. Before this I was completely fine."

She wrote in her notepad and looked up at me. "Hmmm. Well, it sounds like you need to go back on those meds."

Back on the meds? Did you just hear me? I thought angrily.

"No, they were making my heart race. I didn't have the strange thoughts and movements until I *stopped* taking those meds. Before all of this I was fine."

Scott tried to chime in with his assertive tone to back up what I was saying.

She smiled politely, nodding her head at both of us, pretending to listen, but her mind was made up. I was crazy because I stopped taking medication.

"I'll be back shortly," she said.

"I don't think she's even listening to us," I told Scott, furious that she didn't seem to be taking this seriously.

He nodded in agreement.

The social worker returned, and in her bubbly, fake-caring way, presented her recommendations.

"I'm going to send you home. I know you're not feeling good right now. You can keep taking the Ativan like your psychiatrist prescribed until you find the right combination of medications."

My eyes widened. As calmly as I could, I said, "You're not going to keep me?"

"Why would I do that?"

"To see what this thing is. To monitor it. None of this was happening before I started taking these meds."

"But you're functioning," she said.

I was speechless. I couldn't believe what she had just said.

You call this functioning? Functioning is what I was doing before all of this. This is not functioning. I don't know where you were trained, but I'll be sure to never use that phrase with anyone when I become a social worker.

After waiting hours in the ER to be seen by someone only to be told "you're functioning" seemed to diminish the importance of what was happening to me. I was hurt and disappointed that I couldn't get this person to understand why my situation felt so urgent.

I probed for answers. "Can you tell me what's happening?"

"You're probably having a manic episode because you stopped taking your meds."

That didn't make sense. Or did it? Is this what Dr. Pavlichuk meant by opening a Pandora's box? Is this my bipolar coming out? Maybe I was bipolar and this was my manic break. Even though I had feared this happening, something didn't feel right. How does medication trigger a manic episode with bipolar?

"Why can't I stop moving?" I asked her.

"Probably because you're anxious and off your meds." It was clear she had no more time for me.

"I printed out some literature for you to read on bipolar disorder. It might help you understand more about what's happening with you."

"No, I don't need that."

I have spent months researching bipolar. You can take your sheet and shove it.

She passed the sheet to Scott but continued to look at me. "And you should attend our Adult Intensive Outpatient Program. The psychiatrist there is very good. And he can help you find the best medication for you."

Our eyes connected as Scott and I read each other's mind. *There's no way I'm doing that. Clearly, she doesn't know what she's talking about.*

This woman took away the little ounce of hope I had when I went to the ER. All I wanted were some answers, to stop moving, and to not be terrified anymore. Obviously this was not going to be the place for that.

The next couple of days nothing seemed to be getting better. How did I go from sane to crazy so quickly? I had never read that bipolar started like this. I called work and told them I was going to be out for an undetermined amount of time and that I was not in a position to talk, but that Scott would call to keep them informed.

The terror and movements were too much to handle. Scott called friends of his who worked or knew someone who worked in the medical field, but he wound up empty handed. As a last resort, we called my general practitioner to see if I could get in with him to examine me. At the very least, I was hoping he could get me to the next steps. Scott drove me to his office. The three of us had a chat, with Scott and my doctor doing most of the talking.

We all agreed that I needed to be monitored to know more about what was going on. So, that night, at my GP's recommendation, we went to St. Dominic's Hospital and waited in their ER for me to be committed to their psych ward. He called in advance to let them know of my arrival.

Before we stopped off at St. Dominic's, Scott made a pit stop to a friend of his who was an attorney. Scott had some past trauma issues from the Catholic church and dreaded going to one of their institutions. He was also worried that because we were an unmarried gay couple, they might not let him see me. I signed a paper making him my power of attorney.

When we arrived at St. Dominic's, they initially did not want to commit me. That privilege was reserved for those who were suicidal. They had brought me into a padded room, and they made Scott leave. I could hear Scott's assertive tone as he was talking to some staff.

A social worker came in. "Be honest, is he beating you? Is he raping you? We can help you if you're in a domestic violence situation," he said to me.

While this was funny when my friend had asked me years before, I was not having this now.

Are you fucking kidding me? Now I understand why this profession I wanted to enter gets such a bad rap.

"Where did you go to school?" I asked, ignoring his questions.

"I went to Fordham."

Oh, fuck. Is this what they're teaching there? I'm going to have to majorly reassess my career goals when this is over.

"I'm supposed to go there in the fall, and I hope to be doing what you're doing."

He again asked if I was being beaten. "No!" I screamed.

"You seem fine to me."

Why couldn't I convey what was going on with me? I felt like I was speaking a foreign language to people who could not comprehend.

I broke down crying. "I'm not being abused; I'm not being raped. I stopped taking some medication that my psychiatrist prescribed me. I only took it for a few days. He left his practice. A few days later I couldn't stop moving and I'm terrified of everything. I'm scared, I'm frightened, and I don't know what to do."

He seemed unimpressed by my soliloquy.

"But do you want to kill yourself?"

They wouldn't commit me unless I said the magic words. I didn't want to kill myself, but I wanted someone to help me figure this all out, and if that was what it was going to take, then fine.

"Yes, if you let me go, I'm going to kill myself."

He called for some staff members to come and get me. A nurse and a security guard escorted me up in an elevator to a secure locked unit. The security guard made me strip naked, and they took my belongings and put them in a bag. I put on the orange and green hospital clothes that were so paper thin you could tear them if you moved the wrong way. It was so humiliating.

The nurse handed me a pill. "Take this."

"What is it?"

"Just take it," she said, apparently annoyed that I was being admitted at this hour of the night, probably ruining her easy night shift.

She didn't tell me what it was or why I was taking it, but at this point, I didn't care. I took the pill and was escorted to my room. I was greeted in my room by another patient, a police officer who had "anger problems."

"Hey, man. I'm on this side. You're over there," he said with his hands down his pants.

As the nurse left, she said: "The psychiatrist will be here in the morning to see you. If you need anything, come to the front desk. Try and sleep."

I sat on my bed and tried to ignore my roommate, who was watching me while he incessantly masturbated.

"Hey?" he would say, looking at me with his lustful eyes, inviting me to feel him.

Wow, there is something strangely erotic about this and it would make for a great twist on a porn scene. Ugh, I can't believe I'm even thinking that at a time like this.

That night, as my roommate jerked off for about the fifth time, I turned away from him and stared out of the window in my room at St. Dominic's Hospital.

106

How the fuck did I let it come to this?

With no one to get reassurance from, I was berating myself. In my quest to find answers, did I wish this upon myself? Did I just ruin my future? How did I go from a relatively normal person to a psych ward? I pondered all the moments that led to this event and questioned whether I would ever find sanity again. I thought of artists who came before me and went crazy: Pollock, Van Gogh ...

Is this what they felt? Is this how the story goes: I start to go mad now that I finally figure out a path for my life?

Van Gogh really started to piss me off. At least when he was locked up he had a better view. All I had was the brick wall from an adjoining building that blocked the sunlight.

What would happen to me?

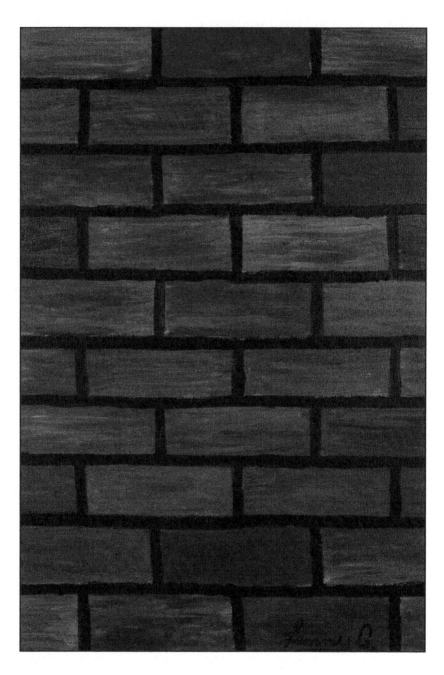

Van Gogh: A Tribute, 2012, oil on canvas, 14" x 18".

CHAPTER 12
"I Feel Great."

The next morning, to my surprise, whatever the nurse had given me had cleared up everything. I wasn't moving and the terror was gone.

Holy shit, it's gone.

I checked my hands. I could keep them still. The sense of terror, not an ounce. Relief flooded my body.

When the staff psychiatrist came to do his rounds, the first question I asked him was, "What on God's earth did you give me? I feel great."

"It was one milligram of Risperdal. Are you still feeling suicidal?"

I never was, but confirmed: "No, I'm not."

The psychiatrist was a straight-to-the-point man. Looking back, I think he might have had some form of autism spectrum disorder. He sat on my bed and asked me to tell him what brought me here. I tried to explain everything up until this point, hoping he would give me some answers. But he couldn't confirm anything, not even the bipolar diagnosis. He really didn't know what to make of the movements and terror and attributed it to anxiety.

"We should keep you for the weekend," he said. I also thought that would be good, just to make sure this pill didn't crap out.

The rest of the weekend I spent with other people struggling with their mental health and some with drug addictions. I attended groups run by nurses, with topics ranging from "the importance of medication compliance" to "how to tie your shoes." Trying not to get called on, I kept my head down in these groups. While I felt safe in the hospital, I couldn't quite connect with the struggles these individuals were facing. Scott came during visiting hours and brought me a piece of onion focaccia from a new restaurant that we both fell in love with months earlier. It was the most exciting part of my day, a moment where I could feel normal.

In a closed room, we sat across from one another, neither one of us knowing what to say. Scott was happy that I was feeling better. "How are they treating you?" he asked, trying to make conversation.

"Okay, I guess."

We attempted to keep things light, but there was this unspoken dialogue that neither of us was saying about what happens next. Now that the crisis was over, we would have to look at the next steps for what this meant for both of us.

After a weekend in the hospital, I was released. Scott came to pick me up. It was a breezy spring day, and being outdoors gave me a sense of optimism.

I was going to have to accept my new life with whatever this thing was that I had. Even though I was feeling better, a tiny part of me knew this wasn't quite over. Edmund was growing inside me, and he would not be tamed so easily.

PART II

"Doctors are men who prescribe medicines
of which they know little,
to cure diseases of which they know less,
in human beings of whom they know nothing."
— Voltaire (1694—1778)

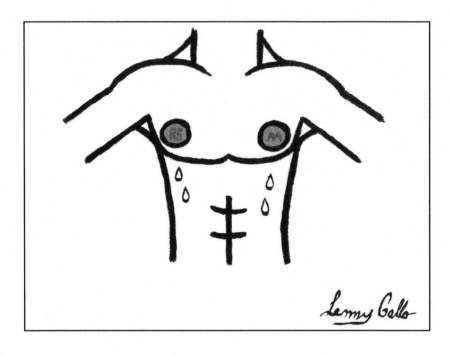

Title Censored Two, 2012, oil on canvas, 14" x 18".

CHAPTER 13

D-Cups

That should have been that. I could go on with my life, right?
The next couple of weeks were a blur. I looked at my discharge paperwork from the hospital, which revealed an unspecified bipolar diagnosis. Even though I wasn't fond of getting confirmation of some type of bipolar disorder, I was feeling better, able to go back to work, and felt I was well on my way to starting graduate school in the fall. Maybe they were right. Maybe I really was bipolar. I worried about it so much, I might as well be.

Feeling good, I thought that we had finally found the right medication that worked for me. I don't know if I ever believed that I could just move on, but it felt like a logical next step. Even though I wasn't paranoid anymore, once you have seen what your brain can do, it paralyzes you; at any point the terror could come back. As I stood outside one afternoon, taking in the fresh air, I kept my eyes from turning toward my car or any others for that matter.

Don't look at them, I silently repeated over and over. I feared that even looking at taillights might set this thing off. The light in the bedroom? Forget it. That shit was covered up with black tape.

Occasionally, I hummed the song that the nurses taught us during one of our group sessions:

Stay on your meds today,

Keep the scaries away.

For the hell of it, I looked up the side effects of Risperdal. It said that it "may cause breasts and lactation in men."

Huh? Wouldn't that be fun! I thought. I seemed to get every other complication from these medications; wouldn't it be great if I got a nice pair of D-cups and started leaking as well? Would save on coffee creamer, and I could tour the world as a *Liza* impersonator. I could take leaky breasts as a tradeoff for my mental health.

Later that week I went back to Dr. Zabel to fill her in on my stint in the hospital.

"I'm still not sure this is bipolar. You don't just have a manic episode come out of the blue, especially after you were on those heavy-duty pills," she said.

"Well, whatever I have, the pills seem to be working well, so I don't care anymore what it is."

She went silent. I could see the hesitant look on her face. She wanted to tell me something but was struggling to say it.

"I was waiting until you were feeling better to tell you this."

Oh no, what? I can't handle anything stressful right now, I thought as I waited for her to proceed.

Her tone had gotten softer, and a look of nervousness overtook her. "I've had to reassess my financial situation," she continued, "and I'm going to be shutting down my practice in a few months. I need to look at my future and my family, and I'm going to have to take a full-time job."

"Oh, no," I said, trying to hold back tears to not dampen what I imagined was a good thing for her. She had helped me so much, and I needed her by my side now more than ever. I couldn't hold back. "What am I going to do without you? I'm happy for you, but . . ."

"I know. I will help you find someone else," she told me, as gently as she could.

I don't want anybody else. I want you.

My fists clenched in an attempt to prevent all of my feelings of hurt from coming out. I'm sure she didn't plan on me having a psychotic break.

Dr. Zabel had been part of private practice prior to the Affordable Care Act. Insurance companies only allowed a certain number of sessions per year. It was a very hard time to be a therapist. You could only see people for ten to twenty sessions, and a lot of patients couldn't afford to pay your full office fee. I understood why she had to take on a more stable job, but the timing felt so wrong.

"We still have this month, so let's at least get you set up with a psychiatrist and therapist you're comfortable with."

About two weeks after my hospitalization, my short-lived success with sanity was coming to an end. Edmund started to reemerge. Once again, the urge to move was relentless, but now I was more attuned to this thing. I would clean the house from top to bottom, go for walks, keep myself busy.

The hospital had referred me to Dr. Manfred. I had a follow-up with him that coming week and decided to mention this to him. As you might expect by now, our interaction didn't go so well.

On our first visit, I told him everything that had happened up until now: "I was doing good in the hospital, but the agitation is back. It's like I can't sit still."

"Let's try you on something else then," he said.

Oh fuck, here we go again.

"Can you tell me what is wrong with me?" I asked as politely as I could, trying to rein in my frustration.

In a cold voice he said, "This is bipolar. You need meds."

Seroquel was next in line. He said that it tended to have fewer side effects. Again, this would not be the answer. After one-quarter of the lowest dose of the pill, my heart started racing, similar to when I was on the Geodon.

I called Dr. Manfred to tell him about the racing heart.

Almost screaming at me, he said, "This is not a side effect that you should call me about."

I didn't respond.

"Stay on the pill or go back on the Risperdal."

"I'm sorry for bothering you," I said, realizing in that moment that I felt nothing.

"You're bipolar, you have to stay on your medication. If you don't stay on this, I'm sending you to outpatient. All medicine has side effects, so get used to it."

No, I don't need to go to outpatient. Why am I not angrier with this guy?

"Okay, I'll go back on the Risperdal," I said, keeping our phone conversation short.

In addition to making my heart race, Seroquel had this strange effect on me where I didn't feel any emotion. I knew I was mad at this guy, but I couldn't feel anger. I couldn't feel happy. I couldn't feel anything.

I tested my heart rate that night the old-fashioned way, and a resting heart rate of one hundred and twenty beats per minute didn't seem like a side effect that was acceptable.

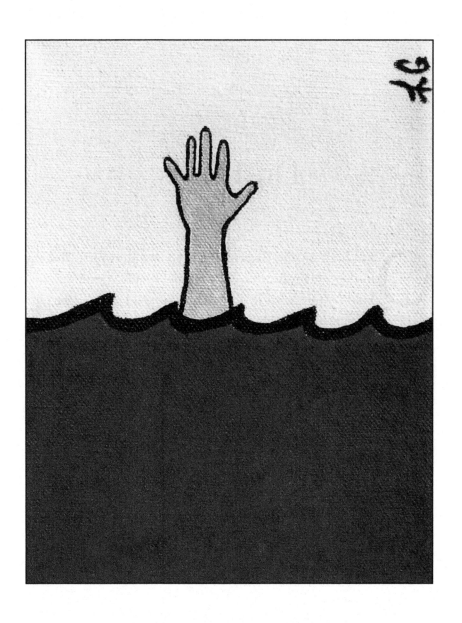

Drowning, 2012, oil on canvas, *6" x 8"*.

CHAPTER 14

Dr. Lewis

Once back on the Risperdal, I felt I was drowning, sinking further and further into oblivion, and I couldn't see a way out. I didn't know what to do, and no one could tell me. The pills were causing so many problems, but I couldn't just stop them, because when I did that, it seemed to make everything worse. The ones that worked only worked for a while, and now these stupid movements and agitation were a part of the equation. Why couldn't anybody tell me what was going on? Clearly, I wasn't the only person who had experienced something like this, was I?

"Will you please listen to me," Nick shouted when I called to fill him in on the current state of things. I was pacing across my balcony, smoking what must have been my fifth cigarette of the hour.

"I checked him out, he doesn't take insurance," I explained.

Nick was persistent. He knew when I was brushing off his comments, and he would get more intense and louder until I got his point.

"You need a *real* psychiatrist. Give him a call."

"I don't know . . ."

He was not taking no or my passivity for an answer.

". . . At this point do you have a choice? You only have a handful of months before you start school. You need to get this shit figured out. Please, trust me, see him."

"I don't know how I'm going to afford this."

"Find a way!" he exclaimed. "This is your health, you've got a husband. You guys will come up with the money."

Nick would never say it to me, but I could sense the anxiety underneath his words. He knew me well enough to know that the state I was in was not me. We were really good friends now. Nick didn't have to speak it, but the tone in his voice often let me know that he was just as scared for me as I was.

I wanted to hang up the phone. We were on the verge of an argument, and I was not in a space where I wanted to debate. Even though I didn't want to hear what Nick was saying, a part of me knew he was right.

To end the conversation, I said, "Let me talk to Scott."

Nick told me about his experience many years earlier with Dr. Lewis and said that he was a great doctor. To be honest, I didn't have any other options. Scott's and my searches didn't uncover anything useful, and I didn't have that long to find a new psychiatrist. If I didn't see him, I was stuck with the man who was ready to put me into an outpatient program.

I called Dr. Lewis' office, and I will never forget the first question I asked his receptionist, "Is he the type of doctor who is going to listen, or is he going to rush me out of there and just give me a pill and send me on my way?"

"He spends a lot of time with his patients," she said, assuring me that I would be heard.

I told her briefly about my situation and why I wanted to come in.

"Let me talk to the doctor and see if he will take you on."

What? Was this like an audition? I thought you just called the psychiatrist and made an appointment. I would have to get pre-approval?

"I'll call you back and let you know what he says," she continued.

I wanted to get another question answered before I let her go. I had to know if this was even going to be feasible. "How much is it per visit?"

"Three hundred dollars for the intake and one hundred fifty dollars for follow-ups."

Could I make this happen? Nick always had the best doctors and could refer you to just about anyone. Later in the day I got a phone call back, and I took Dr. Lewis' next available appointment. Scott and I decided we would at least try this option.

A few days prior, I started to compile a list of everything that occurred since this all started and every medicine I had tried and what happened to me when I took them. At the very least, for three hundred dollars, I wanted answers.

I asked Scott to come with me. If this guy was full of shit, I wanted Scott there to at least be able to call him out like he did with Dr. Pavlichuk.

Dr. Lewis' office, albeit a little retro for my taste with its décor in browns and orange earth tones, was much more inviting than his predecessors' had been. When it was my turn to be seen, Dr. Lewis invited us both into his office and directed us to sit on his couch. Dr. Lewis was the first psychiatrist in this process to smile at me, which, as I had learned, was an unusual trait in the profession. He was an older man, probably my father's age.

"So, what going on?" he asked as he sat down in the chair across from us.

He appeared to be genuinely curious and empathetic, but my guard was up. Ignoring his pleasantries, I immediately went into data giving, detailing my entire story. I was so used to psychiatrists rushing me through the process, my mind tried as hard as it could to squeeze every ounce of information out in the allotted timeframe. When I realized that he wasn't rushing me, however, my body started to loosen. He seemed like he was happy to get as much data as possible and nodded, not in the typical "I'm pretending to listen to you by nodding my head" kind of way, but as if he cared. I handed him my list. He sat there with Scott and me and heard my whole story. I did let myself cry a little as I recounted the horrors of what I had been through with the pills, the psychiatrists, and the hospitals. Scott chimed in with other bits of information, but mostly how much he hated my last psychiatrist and wanted to kill him.

Dr. Lewis sat there, nodding, taking notes, leaning toward us as we provided him with more and more information. With a genuinely empathic smile, he passed me a box of tissues and said, "Thank you for giving me this paper. This is really helpful."

I blew all the snot out of my nose and used that same tissue to dry my eyes. "Do you think I'm bipolar?" I mumbled.

"I don't know," he said in soft tone.

"I just want to get off of all of these medications and get back to where I was before all of this happened."

"You've been through quite a bit," he said, trying to convey that he understood.

I tried to compose myself and asked, "Do you think you can help me?"

Dr. Lewis started to explain what might be going on and what he might be able to do. He believed we could get to the bottom of what was happening and that he could help get me back on track before starting Fordham in the fall. He wasn't sure what to make of the bipolar diagnosis, but since this had been a theme of my medication up until this point, he said we would have to test it.

He calmly went over his plan with Scott and me. Another medication would need to be tried that might help me stabilize better. From there, we could work on getting me off all medications, depending on what happened.

As Scott and I got back into his car, I turned to him and asked: "What did you think of him?"

"I like him a lot better than the last guy you saw."

"I think I do too; he seems to know what he's talking about," I said. I didn't fully trust Dr. Lewis, but his demeanor alone put me at ease. I paused and shifted the conversation. "How will we pay for this?" He wanted to see me again the following week. This was new, as most of my follow-ups were always a month or so away.

"We'll figure it out," said Scott as he was driving away. "We always do."

Maybe I had found someone who was going to work with me to get to the bottom of this rather than just push pills and get me out of there. Time would tell.

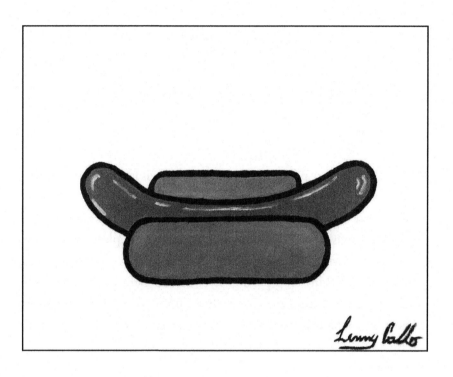

Aluminum Hotdog, 2012, oil on canvas, 9" x 12".

CHAPTER 15
Aluminum Hotdog

The only new pill I ever tried with Dr. Lewis for my mental health was Lithium to help stabilize my possible bipolar disorder so that we could remove the other medication. This was the first part of Dr. Lewis' plan: get me off the Risperdal and replace it with this. I was prone to every side effect, and with Lithium comes frequent urges to urinate. I couldn't stop peeing. Even when there was nothing left in my bladder, the urge was always there. It was like I had a non-stop urinary tract infection. One day, I came very close to peeing my pants during a massage session at work and had to stop the session to go to the bathroom.

The worst side effect of this drug was not the urinary tract infection sensation but the metal taste it constantly left in my mouth. I came home from work one day and made a hotdog for myself for lunch. The whole thing tasted like I was eating a piece of aluminum foil. This aluminum hotdog and my uncontrollable bladder issues were too much. I was not "functioning."

I called Dr. Lewis with the expectation that he would simply tell me to stay on the pill and would be annoyed at what I had done, just like the other psychiatrists. To my surprise, he returned my call in a timely manner and asked me to describe what I was experiencing. Then he told me to stop taking the Lithium and go back on the Risperdal until our next visit.

The following week, Scott and I went to Dr. Lewis' office. Sobbing, I began to hyperventilate and went into full-blown panic attack mode.

"I didn't have any of these problems prior to taking this medication. I don't understand," I wailed.

Trapped in this body that was failing me, it seemed that nothing I was doing would make this stop. I felt incredibly helpless.

I really had hoped that Lithium was going to be the answer, but it wasn't. It was looking like my only options were to be sane and have side effects or go crazy and not be able do much of anything. I kept blaming myself, with Scott and Dr. Lewis watching and trying to calm me down.

"Why did I take those pills?" I wailed. "What did those pills do to my body?"

Dr. Lewis could see my pain. He came over to rub my shoulders and gave me a paper bag. I took the bag, breathed in and out into it, knowing it would do nothing, but feeling reassured by its presence. It was then that he made the decision that had to be made.

He squatted down in front of my chair and looked straight into my eyes, "The only way we're going to get to the bottom of this is to take you off of all of these pills and see what you were like before."

My eyes widened. I could feel my guard come up. I think my heart stopped for a moment. He could see the look of horror on my face. The possibility of experiencing that terror again made my body freeze.

"We have to do it, Len, it's the only way to know what all of this is."

Oh, no, we've already been down that road, and it didn't end well.

As much as I wanted off these pills, was begging to get off them, I didn't want to lose my sanity. I questioned if this man really knew what he was talking about. The only pill he wanted me to stay on was the Ativan, since it would help calm my anxiety and help with the transition.

I looked at Scott to gauge his reaction. He was nodding and seemed to agree with Dr. Lewis. While I wasn't sure I could fully trust Dr. Lewis, I did trust Scott.

I turned toward Dr. Lewis and mentally tried to assess if there was another way.

There was complete silence in the room.

After a few moments, I reflexively blurted out: "I don't want to end up back in a psych ward; I don't want to be afraid."

"I won't let that happen to you."

The starting date for school was fast approaching. I didn't have much time to figure this out.

What could I do? At least this man was willing to work with me and see what was going on. After a few seconds, which seemed to me like forever, I decided to try his plan. What were my other options? Hesitantly I said, "We can do it."

He told me to slowly taper the pills over the course of a few weeks. "If anything happens, you let me know."

It was time to explain to my boss what was going on with me. It was the first time I went into detail about my mental health issues with her. I told her I wasn't sure what was going to happen. She took me off the schedule for a month. If I was feeling better before then, I could call her and have her put me back on, she said.

Scott and I went to Verona Park on June 27, 2012. That morning, I had taken my last bit of Risperdal. I had gotten most of my wish, with the exception of Ativan, I was off all of the pills. Much like when I got off the Geodon, not much happened as I went through the taper. But every day I got up, went outside, looked at my car, and checked to see if the taillights terrified me. It was the only way I knew to gauge my sanity.

"Are you ready for me to go crazy again?" I said to Scott as we sat on a bench looking out at the pond in the middle of the park.

"Stop it, you're going to be fine. Try and be present. You have time off from work, and you can just relax."

You try and relax when your brain is going haywire and there's a possibility of losing touch with reality. Relax? Please! Who could relax at a time like this?

"I feel like a senior who has to be accompanied to the park for my daily outing. Did you bring some bread so we can feed the ducks? Maybe you can take me to get my hair permed after this."

Scott chuckled. "Just enjoy the weather."

That week seemed to be going very well with no pills. No taillights were scaring me, no paranoia. It didn't stop my worry or fear that it might come back. To prove to myself that I was capable, I drove myself to Verona Park on a few occasions. I listened to showtunes on my iPod, one of the few things that still brought me some pleasure. The show of the moment was *Next to Normal*, a story about a woman who was struggling with bipolar and the effect and toll it takes on her family. As I heard the main character, Diana, sing the lyrics to several songs about her battles with mental health and how that broke up the family, the only thing I could think was: *I hope my fate is not yours.*

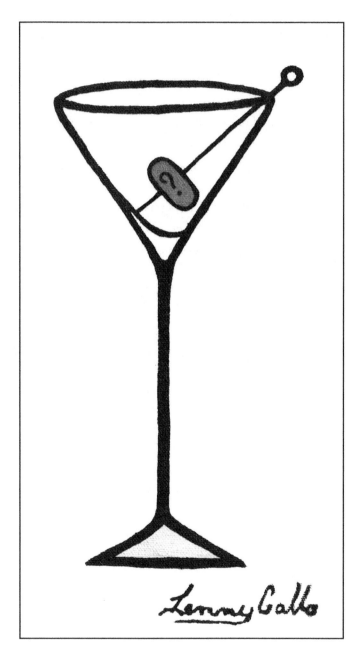

Titled Censored Three, 2012, oil on canvas, 6" x 12".

CHAPTER 16
The Antihistamine

Scott had a friend from out of town, someone also in radio, who wanted to spend some time in New York. It would be during my taper. He would have canceled this visit, considering what was going on with me, but I gave him the green light. Mentally I was feeling the best I had during this whole process and even felt guilty for taking off from work. On July 4th, we celebrated the holiday in New York and went to a Korean BBQ, my first experience with this cuisine. I loved it and wondered why I had been so against trying this in the past. Walking down the streets of Manhattan, with the city's heavy summer air, rats running in and out of the mounds of garbage piled high, inspecting their next meal, and watching the fireworks over the Hudson River, offered a pleasant distraction from all of the chaos that had ensued the months prior. July 5th, however, would give Dr. Lewis the data he was looking for.

That morning I woke up squirming, unable to sit still. I felt an incessant urge to move every muscle in my body. The agitation had returned, only now it was more intense. Periodically, my muscles locked up, almost as if I couldn't move them. There came a point when standing felt too difficult, and all I could do was lie on the floor, squirming. I expected the terror to set in, but this time it did not come. Still, the fear of that made the day even worse.

I called Scott into the bedroom to come check on me. "This is what was happening with Geodon, the movements."

Scott was playing host to his visiting friend but could see the horror of me moving and squirming on the ground. I had him take a video of me to document the experience, just in case.

When I could get it together, I called Dr. Lewis, and he scheduled an appointment for the following day. That night I didn't get a single ounce of sleep.

The next morning Dr. Lewis got to meet Edmund. He could see me in distress and started asking a bunch of questions, almost as if he was assessing me, but his tone soon turned apologetic.

"Oh, Len. I'm sorry this is happening to you," he said.

I was crying hysterically. "Why can't I sit still?"

He talked to me, trying to calm me down. "This is *not* bipolar, this is panic."

What? This was more than a panic attack, I thought, brushing off his comment.

I feared he was going to push this aside as another moment of my anxiety, and that is not what this was.

"What you're experiencing now is panic."

"What about the terror I was experiencing in the nights coming off of Geodon?" I said.

Dr. Lewis asked further questions, and my answers revealed that I was consciously aware throughout the whole process. I wasn't going psychotic like I thought I was.

"If you were psychotic, you wouldn't be aware. You knew it was happening to you," he said. Maybe you had a lucid psychosis. But it feels more like depersonalization and derealization to me."

My body was so revved up, he believed it was detaching from itself. He also believed that coming off the heavy medicine was partially to blame for the feelings of terror I was having.

"So, I'm not bipolar? What about my time on Celexa and some of the other antidepressants? They made my mood worse and made me depressed," I said.

"I'm not sure about that, but it happens with some of these meds. You were probably having paradoxical symptoms. That's not uncommon and doesn't confirm a bipolar diagnosis."

You've got an answer for everything. I like that.

He didn't make me feel stupid for asking questions. The more he listened and talked to me like a human being, the more I opened up.

"Len, I know you don't trust me. The medical system failed you, and I'm sorry about that, but you're not going crazy."

Just hearing that made me feel sane. He was right. I didn't fully trust him. I didn't trust any doctor anymore. None of them seemed to care about what was going on with me, but, for that moment in his office, I trusted him completely.

The big questions, however, remained: What was causing these movements? Why couldn't I sit still?

Dr. Lewis knew that I wanted every question answered and that I needed data and facts.

He went to his bookshelf and dusted off a copy of an early edition of the *Diagnostic and Statistics Manual.*

Great, he's using outdated material. Even I know the DSM has been updated, and I haven't started school yet.

As he thumbed through the manual, he said, "You're having withdrawal akathisia." It was the first time this word had been introduced into my vocabulary, but there was a name for this, which made me curious to know more. "It makes you agitated," he continued. "All of this moving . . . that's what it is."

He handed me the book, pointed out that it should only last about six weeks, and said that we would have to wait it out.

Six weeks? I could handle that.

Scott asked, "Why didn't the other doctors catch this?"

131

Dr. Lewis shook his head and shrugged his shoulders. He didn't want to say that they were incompetent, but his eyes rolling up seemed to infer that.

In addition to the Ativan, he prescribed Diphenhydramine, or as it is more commonly known, Benadryl, and said we should bring back the Trileptal because I had handled that better in the past and it might help with the anxiety until I settled down.

Benadryl? Is this fucker just trying to sedate me? I was angry. *Benadryl?* I did not know that Benadryl was used to treat movement-related disorders, specifically those associated with Parkinson's.

Terrified, I said to Scott and Dr. Lewis, "How am I going to go to work like this?"

"I think you might have to take some time off," Dr. Lewis replied.

I went silent for a moment and distanced myself from the room as my mind turned inward, scrolling through all the data that had just been thrown at me. In that moment, my brain conjured a real fear. "And what about Fordham?"

"You should be fine for the start of the school year, but we're going to have to take it one day at a time," Dr. Lewis said.

Nothing could be done but wait?

I couldn't help but focus on the worst-case scenario. So many life decisions felt like they had to be made that night. He spent an hour trying to calm me down, making sure I understood everything.

Afterward, Scott and I stopped by our local CVS to pick up the Benadryl.

That night, as I moved incessantly, I took my cocktail of drugs with the mysterious Benadryl in the mix. I wasn't one hundred percent convinced that it would solve anything, but it felt like a step in the right direction, and that's all I needed at this point. At the very least, Benadryl gave me a good night's sleep.

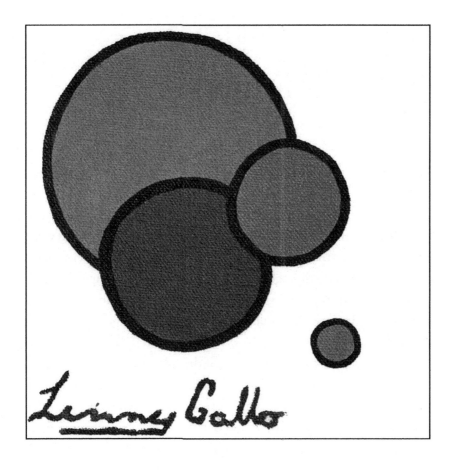

Edmund or Agitation, 2012, oil on canvas, 6" x 6".

CHAPTER 17
Edmund

How do I describe Edmund to you? At first, he was that terror that overwhelmed me. Then he morphed into these movements that were overtaking my body. I wish I had the vocabulary back then to verbalize it. The best way I've been able to tell others what I was feeling was that it was like an agitation and a surge of electricity constantly shooting through me. It's like I drank thirty cups of coffee, but all I wanted to do was go to bed, yet Edmund wouldn't let me sit still for long. For me, this agitation came with tic-like movements, very similar to Tourette's.

Torture is probably a better way of describing Edmund. I wanted to jump out of my skin. If I could have ripped my skin off, I probably would have. Every muscle in my body wanted to contract and move at different times, and I was not being allowed to sit still. I could fight the urges, which I tried many times. Yes, if I tried to consciously focus on an area of my body, I could stop the movements, but all that did was build up Edmund's agitation and make the next set of movements more torturous.

There was not much I could do to try and calm Edmund down. I went for walks around the block to try and get him out of me. I wore my massage scrub bottoms and strolled through the neighborhood at all hours of the day and night. If the neighbors didn't already think I was crazy, well, now I certainly gave them something to see. I must have walked around the block fifty or so times a day trying to tire myself out, but Edmund never tired.

He caused both an external and an internal sense of agitation. It was like an anxiety attack, but ramped up. I tried to breathe and meditate, which sometimes helped, but all I wanted to do was sleep it off, like I would a hangover—but Edmund wouldn't let me sleep. And that's nowhere near the full extent of what Edmund was capable of doing.

Most people find it difficult to understand Edmund, because they often don't have anything to compare it to. If I tell you that I've got the flu, you can relate. If I have a broken bone, even if you've never had one, you know what I'm talking about. We are familiar with those types of illnesses, pain, and discomfort. But how does a person relate to another's inability to control the movements of their body? In general, we don't have a framework for that. The closest comparison is Parkinson's. People have some familiarity with that, but if you tell them it's like Parkinson's, they simply envision you shaking all day with a Parkinsonian tremor, and it's not that at all—it's something quite different. At the time, I didn't know how to describe all of this to my doctors or to the people around me. And now Edmund had gone a step further—he was taking away my ability to work.

I had been working since I was twelve years old, when my dad drove me and a friend to the golf course on weekends, where we caddied for pompous assholes, who had way too much money. I have always felt a sense of pride in my ability to take care of myself, and now, for the first time in my life, I was unable to. In addition to having to figure out how to best manage this movement-related thing, I also had to figure out how I could manage financially. Because of my odd work hours, I wasn't officially able to collect temporary disability, but, luckily, I had signed up for a plan through my massage union that would pay me. It was a mere eight hundred dollars a month, which would barely be enough to cover my bills, but I had no choice. I certainly couldn't present this way at work.

The next handful of weeks I followed up with Dr. Lewis. At each visit he checked to see the intensity of the movements and assess my overall mental health. During this time, I got to know and understand his approach. He wasn't like a typical psychiatrist. He legitimately cared for me and wanted to help. He was able to keep me from drifting too far off into the future and was always able to bring me back to the present. The more I met with Dr. Lewis, the more I felt that Nick had pointed me in the right direction.

We tried other medications in an attempt to lessen my symptoms. Valium, another benzodiazepine, made me want to kill myself. This was followed by Amantadine, a medicine used to treat the flu, but it had an off-label use in the psychiatric world for movements caused by medication. This pill made me nauseous, and I only lasted on it about a week. But the one thing that pill did do for me was take away the internal agitation I was feeling. I would have stayed on it, but I couldn't keep anything down in my stomach.

Six weeks passed, and we entered the final weeks of summer. Edmund showed no sign of letting up.

Why wasn't this thing going away like Dr. Lewis and the DSM had suggested?

The day I had been dreading was fast approaching. My internship placement at Fordham needed to know whether I would be able to attend in the fall. I had been putting them off for as long as I could, telling them I was working through "health issues." But I needed to give them an answer. I talked to the admissions department on the phone. "Hypothetically, if I give up my spot this year, will I be able to attend next year, or will I have to reapply?"

"That depends on why you give up your spot," the woman said.

"For a medical reason," I said.

"We can put you on medical leave for up to a year. You would have to reapply, though."

Fuck. Those applications were not like filling out some form to work at McDonald's. It had taken me months to gather everything for my original application.

"Since you would be on medical leave, however, we would need one more letter of recommendation, which could come from your doctor. You would also have to add an amendment to your essay."

My essay was kick-ass, it was the best thing I'd ever written. Amend it? Who are you?

The woman continued. "The amendment could just talk about how you are feeling better now and what you have learned from taking time off from school."

"So, there wouldn't be a guarantee?"

Don't you want my money? I thought. I had worked so hard for this, and now it felt like I had no choice but to let it go.

"No," she said.

The woman on the phone must have realized that she was stabbing a knife into my heart. She proceeded to say, "We want you here. With a strong recommendation and an amendment, it shouldn't be a problem. Why don't you think it over tonight and let me know tomorrow? I don't want to put any pressure on you, but there are still people who need to be put in field placements, and they could use your spot if you're not going to take it."

I talked it over with Scott and told him there was no way I was going to be able to focus on a graduate program with this going on. I couldn't sit still. How was I going to sit through a full day of lectures and writing papers?

The past couple of years had been spent trying to figure out what the next steps were, and now that I had, my body wasn't going to let me move forward. I was reassured when the admissions woman said that they wanted me at the school, but without a guarantee, the decision was much harder to make.

I thought that entire night. *Could I fight through this? Maybe in a couple more weeks this will be better? Should I just try it and see?*

The answer was no. Edmund was overtaking me.

The next day I called the admissions woman back and made one of the most painful decisions of my life. "I'd like to go on medical leave," I told her, trying to hold back my tears.

"Okay. You take this year to get better. If you're feeling better in January, you can always call back then as well."

That was it, a conversation that lasted less than a minute to undo the work that had taken years. I released my space, and there was no taking that back. Even though this hurt tremendously, there was another part of me that felt a weight lifted off my shoulders. At least now I could truly focus on my health.

A year. That should be enough time to figure this out. Right?

I wanted to believe that this would clear up. In fact, in order for me to accept my decision to let go of Fordham for now, I needed to believe that. In reality, as I reflected on all the preparation I had done over the past couple of years to get to this spot, all I felt was failure as I watched everything being taken away.

Another day that I dreaded was approaching. It was the day of my final appointment with Dr. Zabel. With all the stuff that had been happening, we hadn't worked on finding me a new therapist. I didn't really want a new therapist anyway. I told her about Fordham, and from the look on her face, I could tell that she was feeling the same way I was. She met Edmund and saw the movements and how much pain I was in.

We talked about my time in therapy and next steps.

"Maybe when things settle down you and Scott should talk to a lawyer. This feels like a malpractice case to me." I heard her, but my head was not there. In this entire process, my head never went to that space. I didn't want to sue anybody. I just wanted to go back to work and be able to attend school. This wasn't about money or getting payback. This was about getting my life back.

I had scrounged up enough money to buy her a thank you card. That final time I saw her, I handed it to her. "Can I give you a hug?" I asked, as if at that moment she was the mother I never had. She took me in her arms and gave me the biggest and strongest hug I have ever had.

"You are going to get through this. Believe that you are going to get through this." My snot and tears dripped onto her shoulder.

"Thank you for everything," I said sincerely. You've helped me so much." When it was time to go, I was praying that at the last minute she might change her mind.

After giving up on Fordham and losing my therapist, my mind became hyper focused on getting through this, whatever it was. When the Diphenhydramine/Ativan /Trileptal cocktail wasn't giving relief, Dr. Lewis and I tried a few more medications by themselves. At one point, I was so desperate I begged him to put me back on the Risperdal.

In a sad voice, he said, "Len, I know you're in pain, but that's just not the medicine for you."

"I just can't take this anymore. I want my life back," I told him.

Why wasn't this thing settling down? My mind became obsessed with trying to figure out what was going on in my brain and how to get out of this mess. Was this thing fixable? I had known people who did heavy drugs their entire life. They seemed to make it through. I wondered if I had permanently damaged my brain. At Dr. Lewis' recommendation, I saw a neurologist.

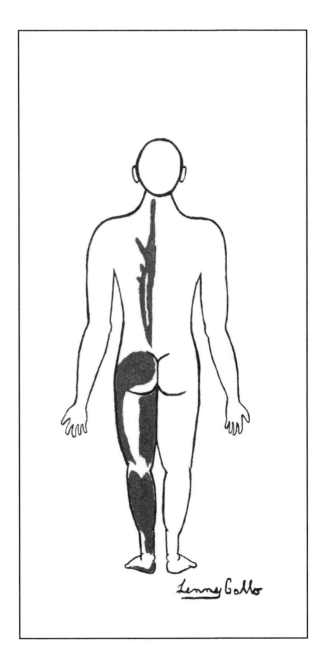

Where Does It Hurt?, 2012, oil on canvas, 18" x 36".

CHAPTER 18
The Neurologist

I was excited to see a neurologist. Not that I did not trust Dr. Lewis—he was the only doctor I did trust at this point. But I felt that it was time for another set of eyes to see what was going on here, preferably not from someone in the mental health realm. Never having seen a neurologist before, I didn't know what to expect. I thought they would run an MRI and see if my brain had been damaged by the medicines.

Dr. Regus appeared to be a crabby old man with a God complex. His office was situated in Closter, New Jersey. It was a sterile place that seemed to have a lot of outdated equipment: parts and machines that looked like they were from a different century. He tried to be friendly at first.

"What's going on, buddy?" he asked in a way that I could tell was put on.

I tried to explain, but about halfway through he cut me off. "This sounds like anxiety . . ."

Fuck, another one of these types. All right, Lenny, give him a shot.

"Well, it definitely sounds like this happened because of the medicine," he added.

That we could both agree on. But he couldn't seem to grasp that my problem was based in my inability to keep still.

Feeling my muscles, he asked, "What kind of pain are you in?"

"I'm not in pain, it's like I can't sit still."

"But you're sitting still now."

"I know, I'm trying not to move."

Subconsciously, I still thought if I forced myself to sit still, Edmund would listen to me.

"Have you done ecstasy?"

What is wrong with you doctors? I'm aware that I shouldn't use drugs. I tried ecstasy once, but that was a long time ago and doesn't seem relevant right now.

I had a very hard time confronting doctors. I wished I had the strength that Scott had to speak his mind. Prior to all of this I always had respect for doctors. I wanted to trust these individuals, but they made it so difficult.

"I tried it once when I was eighteen."

"You know that stuff puts holes in your head," he said warningly.

Seeing that I was getting frustrated, Scott tried to redirect this man back to the fact that everything was fine until the medicine. But Dr. Regus couldn't see it, so to him it didn't exist. Nothing much happened with him during that visit.

On the follow-up visit he kept insisting that there must be some sort of pain, and if there was no pain, then there was no problem. He was God, and what God said went. I didn't have the language to explain my symptoms to him, which only frustrated us both. To test my nervous system, down one side of my body he inserted dozens of tiny needles that shot electrical signals through me. It was like a teenager testing reflexes with electricity on a dead frog in a biology class. The test came back negative, which gave Dr. Regus more conviction that this was all part of my anxiety, a product of my head, and that I should handle my future treatment with Dr. Lewis.

"But why do I keep—"

"You see, the test came back with nothing, so you're fine," he said, interrupting me.

Breathe, just breathe, I thought, trying to keep myself from going full-blown postal on this man.

If I was stronger, I would have argued with this man I so desperately wanted to help me, to give me some guidance, anything. But I had learned that when the medical community made its final verdict, that was it. There was no questioning that verdict. I only saw him a few times. The last time, as Scott and I said goodbye to everyone as we were walking out, Dr. Regus, thinking that we couldn't hear him, mumbled to his staff, "Those two are such a pain in the ass."

Fuck you. You could have at least waited for us to leave the building.

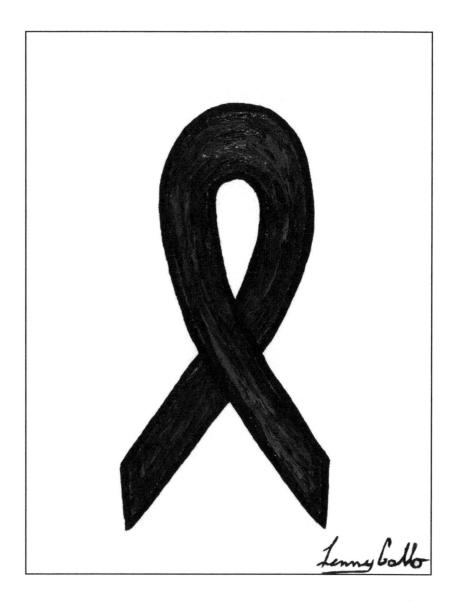

Dystonia Awareness, 2012, oil on canvas, 14" x 18".

CHAPTER 19
Dystonia

Time kept going by and things had hit a standstill. I was anxious, but that wasn't what was causing this. I started to wonder about my future. Would I ever be able to sit still again? Would I be able to sit through a class lecture? I needed answers, and I was not about to give up. If doctors weren't going to help me, I was going to have to do it myself. While pacing and shuffling along throughout the day, I became determined to find out what this was.

I knew that searching my symptoms on the Internet would only give me more anxiety and create more needless fear, but I didn't have a choice. Edmund needed to be understood. And I needed someone who could help me deal with him. It was time to become my own neurologist.

Nothing seemed to make sense about what was going on with me. I was having movement issues, but what kind I could not tell. I would rock back and forth incessantly and try to verse myself in all types of medical terminology and learn about all different types of abnormal movements in the body: choreatic, ataxia, myoclonus, dyskinesia, akathisia, Parkinsonian, and on and on—all these words sounded so foreign. There was researching journal articles, and I did my best to read through these lengthy and wordy documents. I watched YouTube videos on these

145

different types of movements and tried to compare them to movements I was having.

Here was the best I could surmise about Edmund: Based on what Dr. Lewis had said, I had "withdrawal akathisia." Akathisia is a medication-induced movement disorder. It refers to restlessness. It's literally the inability to sit still. It gets divided into three categories: withdrawal, tardive, and chronic. Tardive means delayed in onset. When you start, stop, or change a dose in a psychiatric medication, akathisia can show up. If it shows up days, weeks, or months later, it's considered tardive in nature. Withdrawal akathisia was only supposed to last for about six weeks. This seemed to be the closest to what I was feeling, but why wasn't it going away? Was it chronic? The literature suggested that chronic and tardive forms came about in people who had been on medications for years. I had been on this pill for a week. Even with Risperdal, I wasn't on it for very long. I hadn't really been on any pill long term. It was the closest to what I was feeling, but not the only thing. It was difficult to find any more information on akathisia. Why was mine not going away?

Another medication-induced movement disorder has become more common today, but there was very little information for the average person to find at the time: tardive dyskinesia. This little sucker, much like akathisia, happens while taking, starting, or stopping medication. This condition is where your face and/or body start making irregular, uncontrollable movements. You might start chewing without realizing it or sticking out your tongue without meaning to do so. The movements are slow and polymorphic, meaning that they keep changing their shape.

I had some of those types of movements, but, again, the literature pointed to long term use of antipsychotics. From what I could tell, tardive dyskinesia also seemed to be more localized to the face. Mine was full body.

The truth was, I didn't understand any of what I was researching. My gut was telling me it was closer to tardive, chronic, akathisia, but I couldn't be sure. My movements didn't seem to fit into one specific category, and it became incredibly frustrating not knowing what I was dealing with. And what about that terror I experienced early on? How did that fit into all of this?

One day on my search I found an organization known as the *Dystonia Medical Research Foundation*. Dystonia is an uncontrollable movement disorder by which your body involuntarily contracts muscles for prolonged periods of time.

Hmm . . . this happened to me when I first got off the Risperdal, but it didn't seem to be happening now.

I learned that you could in fact have a dystonic reaction due to a medication withdrawal. I watched more YouTube videos of people who were having dystonic reactions from medication side effects. Their symptoms looked similar to mine, but not completely. Could this be the cause?

I ran it by Dr. Lewis at one of our check-ins.

"Len, you don't have dystonia."

I don't know if I believe you, I thought angrily as he dismissed my research.

"Are you sure?" I responded, trying to keep my feelings to myself.

"People are born with dystonia."

"But you *can* get it from medications."

"Yeah, but that's not what's happening here."

How do you know? You told me this thing would be gone in six weeks and yet here we are.

I know Dr. Lewis was doing his best to keep me calm and stable during this period, but it was torture not knowing where to go or what to do. If I was going to get this thing treated, it was important to know first what I was dealing with.

The *Dystonia Medical Research Foundation* had monthly meetings for people struggling with this disorder. I decided to see for myself and signed up to go to one of their meetings in New York City.

The dystonia meeting was held at Mount Olive Hospital in New York. As I walked into that meeting, I was greeted by many individuals whose body parts were locked in all sorts of positions. Their muscles seemed to contract painfully, with no signs of relief. Some had nothing more than an arm that seemed locked in place, while others had full body contractions that put them into pretzel-like shapes, leaving them bound in wheelchairs. It was one of the saddest things I had ever seen, and I felt incredibly guilty for invading what must have been their sacred space to talk about life with this disorder. I thought about leaving, but the meeting was underway. I decided I would not disturb them and would sit quietly. This was not a quiet meeting, however. Members soon turned their eyes toward me and noticed the new person in the room. Before long, I was getting questions.

"What kind of dystonia do you have?" asked a woman as she pulled up to me in a wheelchair.

"I don't actually know," I told her.

"So, what brought you here?" another said.

I didn't know what to say. I tried to tell them my story. It was a relief to be heard by others and to talk, but I could tell from the puzzled look in people's eyes that they didn't quite know how to respond to me.

I couldn't sit still and was clenching my fists and squirming in my seat. This whole process was so confusing, I started to cry. Where the fuck was I supposed to turn to for answers on this? My tears set off a tidal wave of tears from the other participants, who regaled me with stories of the first time they learned their diagnosis.

Some tried to give me encouragement. "You're going to get through this." A few tried to diagnose me, "This is how mine first started." It was then that Gene, the group's moderator, who had full-blown dystonia, approached. Dystonia had taken her vocal cords, but in what little voice she had, she said, "None of us know what you have, and it's not our place to tell you, but if you want to find answers, you should see a neurologist, one that specializes in *movement disorders.*"

What? Movement specialist? Tell me more.

"We've all been to the neurologists who weren't able to diagnose us because they didn't understand movements. We've all been misdiagnosed and thrown out of doctors' offices because we didn't fit into their box."

I didn't realize that there were subspecialties within neurology. That was it. That's what I needed, a movement specialist.

Everyone was crying again, me included. I thanked Gene for the guidance. While I didn't believe I had full blown dystonia, the one thing I did gain from going to that meeting was the encouragement from all the group participants to find a movement specialist. For the first time in this process, I also got to share my story without anyone invalidating me. That night when I got home and went back to the Internet, I quickly researched movement specialists. Sure enough, there were doctors who came up. This felt like a win. This felt like hope. The next day I made an appointment with the doctors at Cooper Hospital in New Jersey, who had a whole program dedicated to movements.

It felt like I was getting closer to someone who could understand. But nothing in this process was easy. Not a damn thing. Why was everything so fucking difficult? Their program, which had a movement disorder specialty, seemed like a good place to start. But when Scott and I went to that appointment, the doctor had no idea what to make of this. He was much more polite than Dr. Regus and even brought in one of his colleagues to help assess, but neither could make sense of what I was saying.

"Maybe it's your blood pressure," one of them proclaimed. "It is a little high."

Yours would be too if you were going through this.

Scott showed them the video of the July night when I got off Risperdal, but they were inconclusive about what to make of it. I brought up my suspicions about tardive dyskinesia and chronic akathisia, but the response I got was: "We're not as familiar with those disorders."

Apparently, even among movement specialists, there were subspecialties with doctors who focused on movements caused by different things. This program focused more on patients with Parkinson's disease. I wasn't quite sure what I was looking for at this point, but I started to believe that I was really going to need to find a needle in the haystack. The search continued.

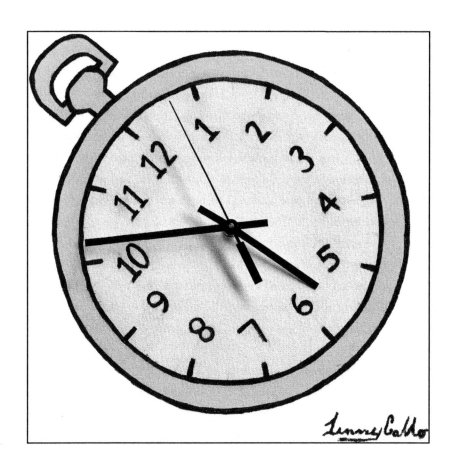

Waiting, Part I, 2012, oil on canvas, 12" x 12".

CHAPTER 20
Waiting

The next phase of my life was the waiting phase that followed visits to different movement specialists. I'll spare you the details of every doctor, but it generally went like this: I would see a doctor, they would tell me they didn't know what was going on, I would move on and wait for the next appointment that would inevitably lead to more useless information. Every time I asked, "But you don't think the medicine might be to blame? What about tardive dyskinesia or akathisia?"

"No, you were never on the medication long enough for any of the stuff you are talking about to happen," many would say. Each time I heard that phrase, it brought me back to the moment when the social worker at Valley Hospital told me I was "functioning." I would turn inward, only to fester more about why it couldn't be that or what else it could be. The discouraging remarks continued to leave me feeling helpless.

What could I say to them? As much as I wanted to scream at every doctor I had come into contact with, I needed to find someone to believe me, understand this thing going on inside of me, and guide me through this process. But all I could do was continue to move uncontrollably and wait. What I wanted to do was sit and watch TV or go to sleep, but Edmund wouldn't have it.

151

Around this time, I turned to my art. As the movements persisted and the accompanying depression started to take over, my drive to find answers and solutions was fading. Much like in my youth, I needed an outlet to let out this frustration. I wanted to write but couldn't concentrate. My brain was exhausted from trying to be my own doctor, worrying, and just trying to keep myself from jumping out of my skin.

Both Scott and Dr. Lewis suggested that maybe it would be a good time to paint or draw. I didn't want to do anything. When you're constantly moving all day, all you can do is focus on when you will stop moving.

Scott drove me to a local art store to pick up a few supplies. When we got home and I looked at those blank canvases, I wanted to pull a Jackson Pollock and just throw paint on the canvas or simply tear them up all together. But, more constructively, I created and painted symbols to depict moments from my current life. I made my compositions in a cartoon style, which felt like a light and uncomplicated way to convey such a complex unknown. Plus, cartoons were one of the few things that always brought me joy. While the figures were simple with minimal detail, the linear work with a black outline required a ton of precision on canvas, and my hands struggled to stay still. I forced myself to complete these works, all while listening to the most depressing showtunes I could find. I needed to feel productive and that I was accomplishing something. To be stuck at home with nothing but my own thoughts made me feel useless.

When I wasn't painting, I spent my time being depressed and moving incessantly. I paced back and forth, trying to watch TV. Sometimes I would plop pillows on the floor and move around on them in front of the TV. Edmund would make me move my feet, compelling me to squeeze them as tightly as possible. Then he would make his way up to my hands and face. The urge to move those muscles became horribly intense as I was forced to do his bidding. I would try and distract myself by watching TV, but often I couldn't even stay with a story before Edmund was telling me it was time to go for a walk. I kept waiting for the day when this would stop, but it never came.

When I was able to follow along with a TV show, it often depressed me. Every time I turned on the TV, I happened to choose a show where the main character was going through some major life crisis. I cried as I watched Monica Porter's character, Kristina, battle cancer in *Parenthood*. Scott walked in on me one day weeping as I watched *Dolphin Tale II*, a movie about a dolphin who loses its tail and needs the help of humans to learn to swim again.

"I'm going to be that dolphin," I told him, sobbing and squiggling on the couch.

I wanted my life back. I didn't want to be like that dolphin. But the pacing and movements persisted.

On another day, Scott asked me as politely as he could, "Do you think a shower would make you feel better?" Bathing and grooming were at the bottom of my list. Days would go by without me showering or brushing my teeth. I was so lost in my head and focused on when the movements would go away, my mind could barely think of anything else, let alone hygiene.

With seemingly no end in sight or answers from the real world, I made prayer another part of my daily rituals. I was not a religious person; Catholic school had ruined that. But Pascal's wager about why one should believe in God came to mind. What did I have to lose? I prayed to Jesus, I prayed to Buddha, I prayed to Allah, I prayed to Vishnu. I was so lost for answers, I even bought myself a deck of tarot cards, hoping to get answers from beyond.

Why did I keep pulling the tower card? It represented the destruction and collapse of everything in one's life.

I asked Scott to drive me to a Catholic church one afternoon.

He looked at me, confused.

"I want to light a candle," I told him keeping the tears inside.

Scott rubbed his head and looked down, trying to contain his feelings. "Really?" he said.

He didn't have to say it; I knew what he was thinking. *"You want to give money to an organization that is blatantly homophobic and that won't even recognize us as a couple?"*

"Yes, really," I told him.

If the medical world wasn't going to help me, maybe it was time to turn to the spiritual. While I shared in Scott's sentiment, I needed something from somewhere.

Scott stared at me, seeing how broken Edmund had made me. For that moment he let go of his anger about the church and recognized that this was about something bigger. This was about giving me hope. Later that day he drove me to the local Catholic church, where I paid a dollar to light a candle.

I was a little pissed off because the church now had fire regulations against unattended candles. They had switched to cheap, battery operated candles, which could be turned on and off by sliding a button. Who the fuck wants to pay a dollar to push a button?

I tried to let go of my anger, however, as I pushed the switch of that candle. I stood looking at the altar's crucifixion of Christ and remember thinking, *I probably shouldn't complain, you seem to have had it worse than me.*

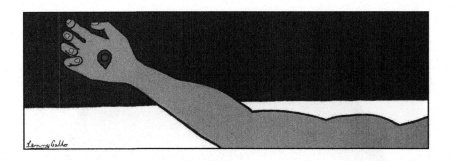

The Crucifixion, 2012, oil on canvas, 12" x 36".

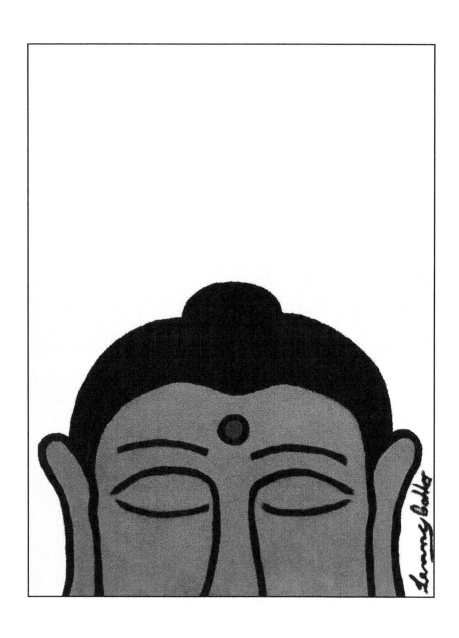

Buddha, 2012, oil on canvas, 9" x 12".

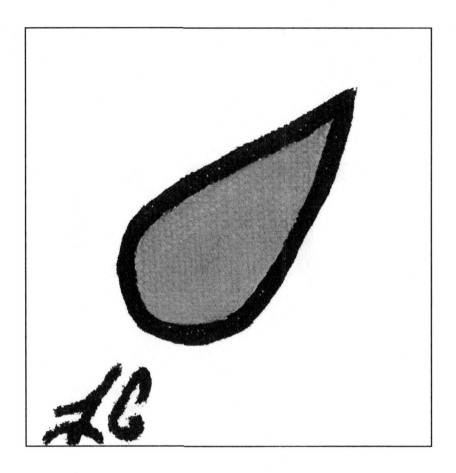

Tears, 2012, oil on canvas, 3"x 3".

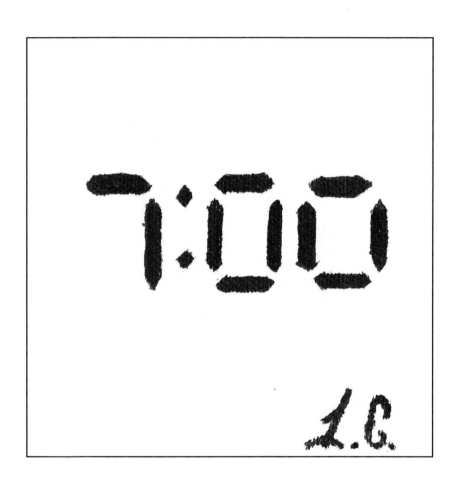

7:00 A.M., 2012, oil on canvas, 3"x 3".

CHAPTER 21
7:00 A.M.

The days blended into each other. I tried my hardest to distract myself and not focus on Edmund, but the only time I would get relief was when I was able to get any sleep. At night, as I would move and squirm and attempt to fall asleep, Scott would hold me in his arms, trying to get me to settle down. I taught him some massage techniques.

He would take his elbow and forearm as best as he could and run them against my thighs while I sat there crying. "Am I going too deep?" he would ask like the good massage therapist I taught him to be. He paid attention not just to my body, but to my emotions as well.

"No, it's good, I'm just sad because this never ends."

In the mornings I woke up always at 7:00 a.m. on the dot. It didn't matter what time I went to bed. Edmund had developed this new alarm clock that I never had before. Always at 7:00 a.m., not 7:01 a.m. or 6:59 a.m. Gone were the days of being able to sleep in as late as I wanted, no matter what time I went to bed or how few hours of sleep I had gotten. I was averaging about three hours a night. There would be one tiny second when I first woke up that I forgot that this whole thing ever happened to me—and then the movements would start back up.

The tears, not caused by Edmund but a byproduct of him torturing me, came pouring out every day. I begged him to stop. I begged Edmund to give me just one ounce of peace. I talked to him as if he could respond: "Will you please just stop? Fucking stop already! Just. Fucking. Stop!" I screamed at my body.

I pleaded and bargained with him. "I'll be a good person, I swear I'll be good." But he never responded in the way I needed. Tears were the first and last thing that came out of my body every day. Edmund didn't care.

My only diversion was when Scott forced me to go out to lunch with him. "I don't want people staring at me," I would argue. "Fuck them, you have to get out of the house."

I was very self-conscious about how people would view me and my movements. Even though when we went out people were usually busy with their own set of issues, it felt like everyone was looking at me.

Before all this happened, we never got to spend time with each other during the day. I would usually be at work. Now we were able to take weekday trips to Costco or the grocery store. On our way home we always stopped at Chipotle for lunch. As I attempted to sit still and eat my burrito, I often asked Scott what he thought about all of this. "It's just sad. I hate seeing you like this, and I hate that there's nothing I can do," he would say.

I never knew what was going on in his mind. I was the younger of the two of us, and when we started our life together, I'll bet he never thought he would have to be the caregiver. At this point it looked like he would wipe my ass before I wiped his.

Being lost in my head all day was not a good thing for me. Scott and Dr. Lewis thought it would be a good idea to get away for a bit. Being cooped up in the house kept me in a festering loop that would go on for days. As a way of trying to get me out of my element, Scott booked us a weekend trip to the Poconos.

"Why are we going, I won't be able to do anything?" I said, dismissing this idea.

"It's just to get away."

I didn't want to go, and my tone of voice indicated my frustration at Scott. "I'm just going to move; what's the point?"

Ignoring my discontent, he said, "Well, then you can move in a different environment."

The weekend was about what I expected, but even if I wasn't at my best, it was nice to move somewhere else. At least there were more trees and nature.

As we drove home from that weekend, Scott sat in silence, and I squirmed in silence. What was there left to say? He was focusing on the road, and I was staring out the window, trying to admire the beauty of Pennsylvania as we drove down I-80 East. I thought about the very first time Scott and I had driven down this road when I first moved to New Jersey. And then the image came to mind that had been pushed back since Edmund had entered our lives: the day I walked into Scott's office and unleashed my feelings on him. I had to do it, but none of that seemed to matter anymore. It all felt so trivial.

I started to reflect on the entirety of my relationship with Scott, all the years we had been together.

Since Edmund entered my life, we hadn't really talked about us as a couple. Everything was consumed with getting me better. As we were driving, I looked at his big brown eyes, much the way I had looked at him the night we went on our first date. I sat there thinking about all he had done for me, and I felt a sense of guilt for bringing Edmund into our lives and not appreciating Scott's efforts, not just now but from the beginning. He had always thought of me and ways to improve our life together—even if I didn't always agree with his way of going about it.

Scott's strong demeanor was a blessing. He helped me survive during this ordeal. He was there for every doctor's appointment; he was there every time I had a meltdown. The truth is, he had always been there. I was just so consumed by my anxiety to ever notice.

I looked at Scott, grabbed his thigh and muttered, "I'm sorry."

"For what?" he said, glancing at me, taking his eyes off the road for a moment.

"For everything," I said, trying to nudge his memory of what our life looked like before this.

"Stop it," he said, as if he had already moved on from that time. But I could tell that he had understood my meaning.

"No, I'm *really* sorry," I said in the most genuine tone I had in me. My eyes began to water up. "I love you, and I couldn't imagine going through this with anyone but you. There's no one else I want to be with, and I'm sorry that I'm saying this to you now, when I'm at my weakest."

I told him how I hadn't always appreciated the role he played in my life and that I was sorry for taking him for granted. A tear fell from his eye, and he told me that he was sorry as well.

Even though I would have never wished Edmund into my life, a positive side effect of this disorder was that it made us grow closer as a couple. We made the choice to work together. It enabled us to appreciate what it really meant to be with each other. This was what real love was about: having someone there in your time of need. It was something I rarely got to experience in my life. Scott had proven that he would be there no matter what. I no longer had doubts about our relationship, and I didn't doubt the love I felt for him. I knew that I would always be with him and that moving forward we would be there for each other.

The rest of the ride home, we talked about everything. Nothing was off limits. I apologized for being so hard on him about buying the house out in the burbs, the tour, and that time he moved out to Los Angeles. He, in turn, apologized for not always listening. Enough time had passed where we were able to distance ourselves from our past reality and objectively reassess our lives together and what we meant to each other. We weren't just talking at each other that night—we both really heard each other, and we made a vow to continue to work on our relationship to build a stronger unit, whatever the outcome of this disorder would be.

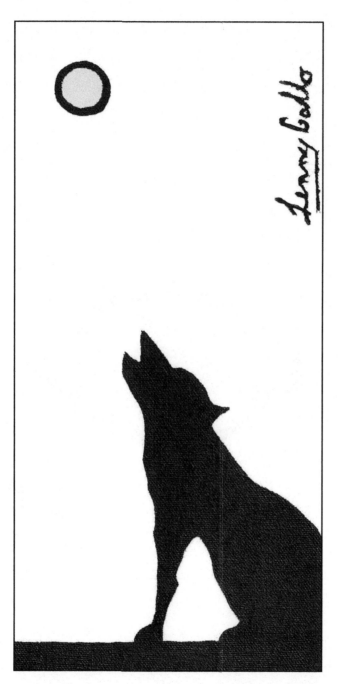

Boy Who Cried Wolf, 2012, oil on canvas, 6" x 12"

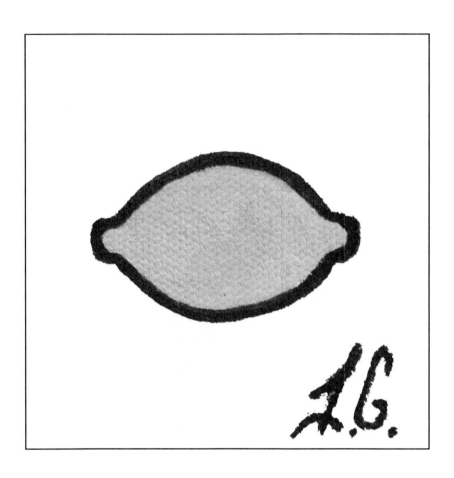

When Life Gives You Lemons . . . or Bitter Fruit, 2012, oil on canvas, 3"x 3".

CHAPTER 22
Friends

My friend Nick and I talked every day. He would call, and he always started our phone conversations happy and enthusiastically: "Are you better today?" Or, "Any improvements?" Frustrated that I couldn't give him new information, but also relieved that someone cared, I would tell him the same thing every day: "No, I'm still the same," I said in a solemn tone.

He never really knew what to say to me after that but tried to cheer me up by keeping the conversations light.

"Are you jerking off at least . . . I mean with the shaking. Scott must love that."

I wished I could have had sex, but my mind wasn't in that space.

I also talked to friends back in Chicago, hoping to get support from them. But the dynamic of our friendships had changed, and I noticed after a while I was starting to wear thin on a lot of them. Some of my closest friends tried their best to understand what was happening to me, and gave as much support as they could, but without actually seeing it, it was hard for them to envision what this was doing to me. Everyone who did talk to me would offer clichéd bits of positivity. It's not helpful when you're going through something that even you don't understand.

You've heard these remarks:

"Everything happens for a reason,"

"Time heals all wounds,"

"It could be worse,"

"What doesn't kill you, makes you stronger,"

 "When life gives you lemons . . ."

This is known as toxic positivity, because, while well intentioned, it underrates a person's pain.

I also got people who offered every bit of wisdom they had: "Have you tried . . ."

What was I supposed to think and feel hearing these things? I felt angry. I didn't want to, but that was the only emotion that seemed to fit. I think that a lot of people struggle to hear you talking about your pain, because it makes them feel helpless, too. I know all of my friends' intentions were good, but it was hard to see that in the midst of all of this. What I wanted was something that didn't exist: another person like me who felt exactly what I was feeling.

Some friends didn't even bother to call. Many were wrapped up with their own lives, I imagined. It's often been said that during trying times you find out who your real friends are. That was certainly true for me. But more than the movements and pacing, more than the fear and terror of the unknown, and more than the toxic-positivity people and people who didn't call, were all the people who implied: "I don't believe you."

Seeing so many doctors with no answers made me feel like a Munchausen patient, someone who is making up their symptoms for attention, or a conspiracy theorist who won't accept the facts in front of them.

At this point I sort of expected doctors not to believe me. What I did not expect was to hear this from friends. What hurt the most was when friends started questioning how authentic this thing was. No one said it outright, but the underlying tone and insinuations behind their passive aggressive words said it all: "This is all in your head."

Clearly, this *was* all in my head, but what the fuck was causing it? Why could no one understand that this wasn't one of my anxious attacks? What was it going to take for me to get people to see? But how could I blame them? When you have spent your life struggling with anxiety, you have a natural tendency to turn many elements of your life into catastrophes. All too often, I was the boy who cried wolf, making mountains out of molehills and expecting the worst to happen. This time there really was a wolf.

I shut down and stopped talking to all but a few select friends, and for the first time I started to lose any hope that this would get better. I was blaming doctors for my pain. I cursed pharmaceutical companies for putting those medications out into the world. I blamed everyone and everything that came into my path.

When cursing others didn't take the feelings of anger away, I turned my attention inward, festering and beating myself up: I pulled my hair out and slapped myself, as if this would torture the insidious Edmund and beat him out of me. And I asked myself the same questions: *Why did I take those stupid pills? Why didn't I listen to my therapist? Why didn't I listen to myself? Would I ever be able to sit through a Broadway show again? Would I ever be on stage again? Did I ruin our lives? Why am I so stupid?* I didn't know if life was going to turn this shit into lemonade, but I could definitely taste the bitterness of that fruit.

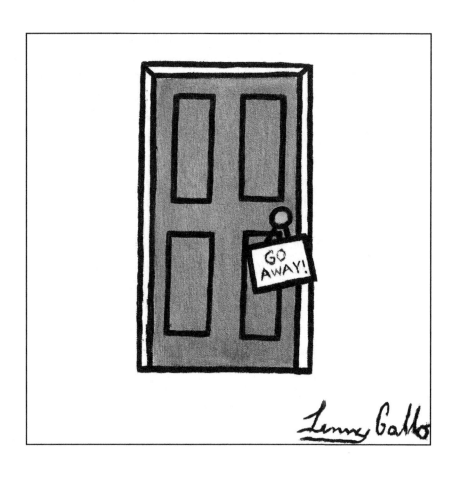

Go Away, 2012, oil on canvas, 12" x 12".

Untitled, 2013, oil on canvas, 18" x 36".

CHAPTER 23

Unstill

"Len, do you need me to come up?" my father asked one day on the phone as I cried while giving him a rundown of my day. My dad and I talked at least once a week. In the years since he divorced my mother, he had remarried and moved to the suburbs of Chicago. He seemed happier and was enjoying life more.

"No, Dad, you don't have to come. Scott is taking care of me." I wanted him to come up so badly. I wanted to hug him. He had been there so much for me in my life, and this was a time when it felt like I really needed him more than ever. I wanted him to say, "I'm coming anyway." I wanted him to see through the subtext of my words. But another part of me didn't want him to see me like this. I didn't want anyone to see me like this. What could he do? What could anyone do but watch me cry and move. Looking back, maybe I needed that: more people to see and share my pain. I wanted him to believe I was strong and that he had raised a child who was capable of taking care of themselves on their own, but he trusted my judgment and what I told him, and he held off on coming.

My mother got wind of what was happening. I knew that someone would eventually tell her. I wasn't quite sure who it was, but my best guess was that it was my brother. He and she still talked semi-regularly.

Prior to all of this, the relationship between my mother and me had reached a vicious cycle of poor communication. It always went like this: We would talk on the phone and keep things light. Then, several days or weeks later, she would call and get mad and scream that I was an "awful son," that I "didn't care about her." I listened to her screaming and tried to calm her down, always asking myself why I was putting up with this. Several weeks later, I would generally get a handwritten or typed letter from her telling me all the things I had ever done in life that were wrong. The times I responded to these letters to tell her how she made me feel prompted further letters from her, in which she would take my feelings and throw them back at me. My mother had sent me one of these nasty letters just a few weeks prior to this whole thing starting. I decided to turn them into one of my art pieces. (I had to blur out the letters, but take a look at *Mom's Bad Genes*.)

Checking my phone one afternoon, I saw a missed call from her. I listened to the message. "Hi, Len, it's Mom. I heard you're going through something out in New Jersey. Give me a call back, I'm worried about you." Just listening to her fake pleasantries made me cringe. But I took the bait. I always fell for it. It was as if my brain had forgotten all of the things that happened months and years prior and by her leaving this nonthreatening greeting, we had a clean slate. This is how she sucked me in. There was no acknowledgment of any previous fighting, just a simple, pleasant greeting. But I always thought that maybe it would be different; maybe this time, she would actually care.

Before I called her back, I ran it by Scott. I always ran my decisions to call her by him because he was an outsider in this feud. "Are you sure you want to do this?" he said hesitantly. "I know she's your mother, but . . ."

"I know. I just feel bad cutting all ties with her. She has no one but my brother."

"Okay," he told me warningly, almost knowing where this would go. "Are you sure you're in the right headspace for this?"

Probably not, but I felt it was best to get it over with. I dialed her number. "Hey, Mom."

Pretending as if she was legitimately concerned, she said, "I heard from your brother that something was going on with you."

I knew it was him.

I kept my guard up. "Yeah, things aren't so good."

"What happened?" she said in a caring way.

Don't take the bait, don't take the bait.

"I had some issues caused by this medicine I was on." I told her all about what was happening, and she listened. For a moment I let my guard down and even allowed myself to cry.

But her callus tone came through almost immediately: "Well, I'm sorry to hear you're going through that."

As if I had said nothing, the conversation immediately shifted to her. These pleasantries were always a vehicle for her to get her needs met through me. "I'm not doing so good either. Your father's alimony checks will be running out soon and I don't know what I'm going to do."

On and on she went as I paced back and forth. I was numb to it. If I were in a stronger space, I would have told her, "Did you hear anything I just said, are you that self-absorbed?"

Breathe, I kept thinking to myself, trying to inhale and calm myself down. Soon it would be over, and I would have fulfilled my obligatory duties as a son.

She never came back to me in the conversation. When I got off the phone with her that day, I realized something about myself and why I connected so much with art and theatre. She never saw me. She never heard me. By doing my art and theatre, I think a younger subconscious version of myself was trying to get her to see me, but she couldn't. Someday I would be able to explore that more, but for now, the pacing and moving continued.

UNSTILL

Unstill and lost in this torture, I questioned whether I would ever find tranquility again; whether I would ever find stillness again. As I sat there moving incessantly throughout the days, the rage would progressively build. Disconnecting myself from almost everyone and everything, for the first time in my life I truly felt as though I was alone in this battle, and I really had no one to blame but myself.

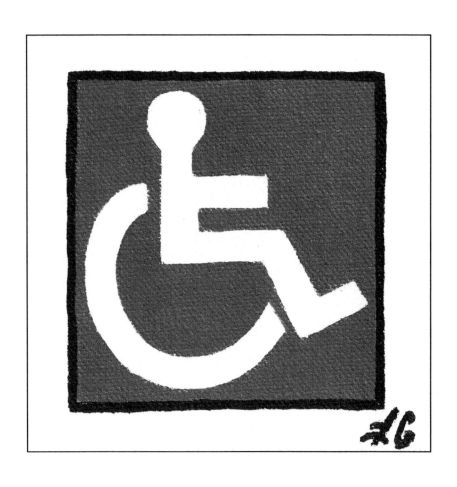

Handicap, 2013, oil on canvas, 4" x 4".

CHAPTER 24

Dependent

My hopes of this ever resolving diminished with each day. If this was going to be a permanent fixture in my life, what would that look like? Was I really going to be dependent on Scott for the rest of my life and have him be my caregiver?

During one of my appointments with Dr. Lewis I brought up the topic. "I think we need to start looking at a more long-term disability," I told him, resolved that this was the state of my life now.

He didn't even flinch. "Disability is for people who don't want to get better and don't want to find a way to be in society again. Why would I want to work with someone who doesn't want to get better?"

Because . . . Because . . . Ahhh, go fuck yourself, Dr. Lewis.

He was always trying to get me to accept my situation and find a way forward, but I wasn't having it. How long was I supposed to wait before I gave up? But nobody wanted to hear it.

I paced my way into Scott's office another day and tried to gauge his mood. Maybe he would go down the rabbit hole with me. Locked away at the computer with his headphones, he looked up at me for a moment. That was the only cue I needed to engage. "Scott, what if this never stops?" We've had this conversation before,

175

but the urgency of the movements made my question feel even more important.

He gave me an exasperated, "Don't go there. This is going to get better."

"No, but what if I can't go to school or work?"

"I wish you wouldn't go there," he said, rolling his eyes at me.

"Why can't we ever go there? When am I allowed to start going there?" I shouted before storming out of his office.

"Please stop putting that energy out there," he said softly, stopping me by grabbing me into his arms. "Give me a hug."

I broke down crying in his arms.

He squeezed me tight, telling me: "You're going to get through this."

Scott was my lifeline. He was the only one who really saw this thing in all its power through every step of the process. Even though we were in a better space, I always feared he would get sick of my health issues and ship me back to Chicago. I dropped it for that day.

When Scott wouldn't give in to my fears, I would call Nick. "Maybe I can be one of those webcam models who jerks off in front of the computer," I told him one day, somewhat serious. I always wondered what that would have been like and how people had the courage to do it.

"They seem to make a lot of money." I could tell by the clanging pots that Nick was making dinner and half listening to what I was saying.

"Right! And there's got to be people out there with a fetish for this shit. Have you seen some of the guys on those sites?"

"Mom," he shouted to the side of the phone, "Do you want a salad with dinner?" He came back to the conversation, trying to wrap things up quickly. "You're going to be fine, just hang in there."

"Yeah, I guess."

Nobody seemed to want to go down this road with me. How did they know I was going to get better? How did they know this was going to pass? Why wouldn't they even entertain the idea? I wanted to plan for the worst-case scenario, but that wasn't going to happen with the people in my life.

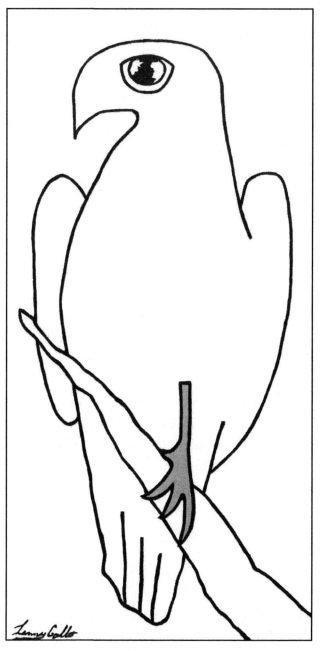

Hope, 2012, oil on canvas, 15" x 30".

CHAPTER 25
The Falcon

I remember the day that an ounce of hope came back into my life. I was pacing outside, smoking on my balcony, as I did every day now. Our balcony sat at the level of the tree juncture, where it makes the V shape. Lost in thought, I heard what sounded like a tree branch fall from a higher limb on one of the many trees that need to be torn down on our property.

I moved closer to the balcony edge to see what had fallen. As I looked down, the supposed tree branch came flying back up at me! It was a falcon that had perched itself on a limb just below where I was. This was a very rare thing to encounter. I held my cigarette tightly. I was scared, shocked, and jumped back as far away as I could. I wasn't sure what this bird would do. My heart raced when I realized that I was now in a spot on the balcony where I could not access my door without passing the motionless bird.

"Go . . . get away," I said to the falcon, as if it could understand. It turned its head toward me. I took a hit of my cigarette and tried to scare it away by blowing smoke at it, but the falcon did not move. It sat there looking at me, unafraid. As I scanned the bird with my eyes,

I noticed that it only had one of its claws, but it didn't seem to be in pain. *Was I in danger? Could birds get rabies?* I wondered.

The bird started pecking with its beak at the area around its amputated claw as if directing me to pay attention to it. When I realized that the bird was not doing anything to me, I calmed down slightly. Still guarded but loosening up, I stared at that bird for what seemed like an eternity. I thought about how hard it must be for this creature to survive in the wild. And I thought about the last time it might have eaten. Teardrops started rolling down my face. My fear soon turned to compassion and a different type of energy overtook me in that moment—one of connection. Its amputated claw resonated with me, and my heart broke for this creature. If this bird, which needs its claws to survive in the wild, can thrive with just one and do that alone, then surely I could survive with whatever the hell was happening to me. As I inched toward the bird, to see how close I could get to this disabled creature, it sensed my movement and flew off. But the feeling it had triggered stayed with me. I made a choice at that moment to keep fighting and vowed to see this thing with Edmund through.

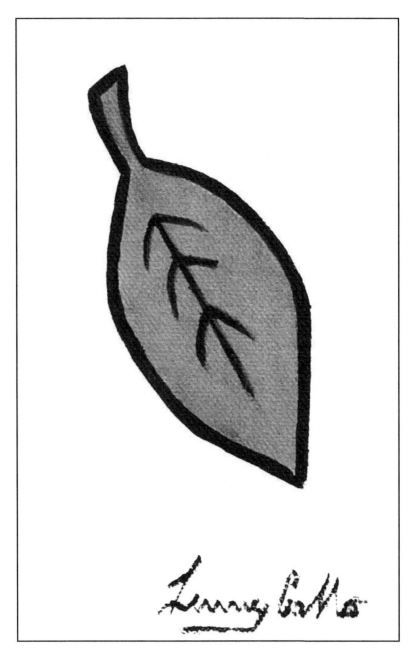

Fall, 2012, oil on canvas, 4"x 6".

CHAPTER 26
Fall

Something different happened when the leaves started to change and the weather got colder. My routine was the same, but after being jolted out of bed one morning, I noticed that my body wasn't moving out of control all day. I could actually sit in a chair without rocking back and forth.

This is new, I thought with some excitement, but cautious about what it meant. As quickly as it came, it went away. But for that one brief time, I felt free from this thing. It was the first time I got a glimmer of what my life was like before Edmund had entered it. Soon, another moment like this came out of the blue. And then another. The periods of not moving happened more frequently throughout the day, and my movements started to decrease in intensity.

When the movements settled down, I felt brief moments of peace, but in a way it was more upsetting than having Edmund torture me all day. During the pauses, I let myself believe I was getting better, only to be reminded of the torture moments later when the movements returned.

But this wasn't all a fluke. Edmund was losing steam. The more days that went by, the more Edmund would settle, and I felt his intensity lessen. Edmund almost always dominated my morning, but by the afternoon I could get as much as a couple of hours free from him. He then came back at night. Some days his waxing and waning would be sporadic: whenever he felt like it, he threw me curve balls. Tears fell every time he decided to remind me of his presence, almost as if he was torturing me in a different way. "Fooled ya! You thought I was done with you? I was just taking a nap."

Others noticed the decrease in Edmund as well. "Today seems like an easier day for you," Scott would say to me, hoping I was in the mood to hear that. He observed that my body could sit through a meal, and I seemed to not move as much.

"Yeah, maybe," I told him.

When I visited Dr. Lewis, he would observe my body and say: "Look, you're all better."

"Uh, no," I told him, not believing for one second that this thing was over.

Even Nick, who hadn't actually seen me during the whole process, noticed that the tone of my voice had changed, sounded more upbeat.

As more and more of these moments occurred, my body started to get some drive back into it.

Things were changing. Waiting seemed to have been paying off. As the days passed, I was able to do more on my own. I started cooking simple meals. When it was time to see Dr. Lewis, I went to some of my appointments on my own. My constant movements were turning more into episodes that would come and go throughout the day. I felt well enough to start driving locally. Sometimes I would make it through a whole TV show without having to get up and down from the couch.

Even though I was better in some respects, and some of the movements were settling down, I still didn't feel like myself. My mind remained lost in this obsessive loop of what had transpired. When you have gone to places you never thought your mind could go, you start to not believe in the little wins that you are getting. How could I trust that my body was actually getting better? And what was it getting better from? I was too afraid to accept these moments as signs of improvement, because I still hadn't gotten much in the way of answers.

The insurance company that was paying for my sick leave gave me a call one day. The person's tone sounded pleasant and nice. "Hi, Lenny, this is Tim from Hetfield Insurance. I just want to check on you."

"Thanks, Tim. I'm getting there," I said, thinking that he was concerned.

"You're on a recorded line by the way . . . That's good to hear. Really good. I'm sure you're dying to get back to work. Must be hard being home all day. What if we pay for a gym membership for the year and get you to get out again? Would you feel comfortable going back to work?"

All I've been doing is moving for the past five months, and you want to pay for me to go to a place so I move even more? I was annoyed and pissed that I had answered the phone.

"I still haven't been able to get a diagnosis on what's going on," I told him.

"That's how these things are sometimes. We don't always know what they are, but we have to get back to work. Get back into life." He sounded like a salesman, but I wasn't buying his bullshit.

I was not about to let this man push me back to work without getting some kind of confirmation on what I was dealing with. This wasn't a broken leg. It was quite clear this man had no idea of what he was talking about.

Coldly, I told him, "I think I would rather wait."

"What would it take to get you back to work?" I understood Tim's point of view. I was a young man and the insurance company thought I was going to follow the statistical trends and not give them a problem. They wanted to save money.

"Maybe I should at least get a diagnosis and let this settle a bit more," I told him. The truth was, I couldn't go back to work at that time. Although I was getting better, Edmund was becoming unpredictable. I would have moments where I was doing fine, but others where I would be pacing again. I could never predict what my body was going to do at any given moment. It would come and go when it pleased. I wasn't moving 24/7 anymore, and I wasn't in a state of constant terror, but the seeds of trauma that had been implanted in my head sprouted every time Edmund came to greet me. The slightest movements would trigger me and put me in a space that made me think that I was back at square one. I didn't feel comfortable doing anything beyond the basics until I knew exactly what it was I was dealing with.

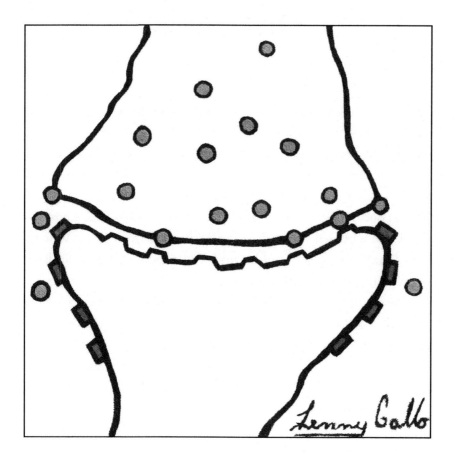

The Verdict?, 2013, oil on canvas, 10" x 10".

CHAPTER 27

Dr. Kurtis

By the time February 2013 came around I finally got an appointment with my next neurologist, Dr. Kurtis. I drove myself. I was doing well enough, and I didn't think I would need Scott there, because I thought this was going to be another round of doctors who would provide useless information and I would be on my way. This was also a difficult doctor to go see, because he was affiliated with the same hospital that I was supposed to intern at for Fordham the year prior. When I signed in, I picked up one of his cards and noticed that he specialized in psychiatry and movement disorders.

Interesting. That seemed like a very odd and specific specialty. I almost allowed myself to get excited but kept my reserve. Experience taught me that nothing came easy. Thirty minutes had passed waiting for this man, and I wanted to leave. Sitting in chairs for too long agitated Edmund.

When finally I was called in, an older man with a very friendly smile greeted me. He appeared to have a bit of a movement disorder himself as I noticed a slight shake and tremor in his hand.

"How are you doing?" he asked.

"Ugh . . . I don't know where to begin," I said.

I wasn't in the mood to go over all of this again. Intakes were hard, because you had to keep repeating yourself over and over.

Unfazed by my guardedness, he probed in a genuinely curious tone:

"How about we just start at the beginning?"

Hesitantly, I opened up and started to tell my story again, for what seemed like the millionth time, but as I was talking, he did something very different than the other neurologists. He asked questions, very specific and well thought out questions. I could tell he wasn't asking these questions to try and fit me into a mold, but rather to form a hypothesis from what I was telling him.

"And when did you start taking that pill?" he would ask.

He wanted to know all of this? Genuinely know?

"And what was the reason for this pill?" he asked. It seemed that he wanted to know every pill I had ever been on. I was happy to give him every bit of data I had in me. He listened to everything, and I even started to throw out terminology that I had learned from all my research.

"It sounds like you know more than most neurologists," he said to me.

Well, I don't have a PhD in this, but if researching the Internet can give me an honorary doctorate, I'll take it. Lord knows I probably just threw away my chance at Fordham.

Dr. Kurtis did all the usual stuff that movement disorder specialists did. He had me touch my nose with my index finger. He tested my reflexes and bopped that rubber thing on my knees. He even gave me a pseudo-sobriety test, making me walk on an imaginary tightrope, one foot in front of the other, trying to balance myself. What was different was that he took the time to do one of the most thorough intakes I had ever had. He sat and listened to my story in its entirety and didn't rush me. And he took insurance. I couldn't believe it.

After all the questioning and analysis, it was time for a verdict.

"Well, I have a theory," he said.

While he couldn't say for sure exactly what was going on with me, he certainly had more ideas than all the preceding neurologists. Dr. Kurtis suspected tardive dyskinesia.

"I thought you had to be on the medication for years in order for that to happen," I said to him. Tardive dyskinesia was associated with individuals who had been on antipsychotics for a long time. The people who got tardive dyskinesia also were on old-school antipsychotics. Think of the olden days when they would lock up people in a "sanitarium" and pump them full of medicines. These medicines were early antipsychotics that caused myriad problems. I ruled this out early on based on my YouTube assessment.

"It's becoming more common than you think, and sometimes it doesn't have the standard movements that we expect. We're seeing it more and more in newer antipsychotics as well and with people that haven't been on them that long."

My jaw dropped. Was this man actually taking me seriously?

"You may have been on these types of meds longer than you think. Whatever this is, it all probably started years ago when you were taking Reglan. Geodon probably set it off."

This was the first time I learned that the wonderful stomach pill I took years prior worked on the brain much like an antipsychotic. He wasn't wrong. A web search revealed that individuals were in the process of going through a class action lawsuit against the makers of Reglan because they had gotten movement-related issues from that pill. While I wasn't on any antipsychotic that long, I had been on Reglan on-and-off for a while, which did very similar things to the brain.

So many emotions were running through me, I could barely keep myself together. I was mad that I took Reglan, but happy that this man was listening to me. I was sad at how long it took to get to this moment. I wanted to scream at all those other fucking doctors, and say, "I told you so," but I kept my composure, because what I really wanted was to hear more from this man. He explained what he thought was going on in my brain, and he even drew me a diagram that I could take home with me. His theory had something to do with my dopamine receptors.

"These medicines that you were on block the dopamine receptors," he told me. That much I understood from my research. He continued, "Dopamine is partially responsible for movement. What we think happens is that when some people take antipsychotics or Reglan, their brains start forming new receptors in response to the medicine blocking their receptors. These new receptors become hypersensitive, and these hypersensitive extra receptors give you the extra movements. When you remove the medication . . . "

"You have a lot of receptors working," I finished for him. I paused for a moment and then asked, "But what about some of the other stuff? The terror and the agitation?"

"It's all probably related to those receptors, but I can't say for sure. The brain is incredibly complex."

By the time I saw Dr. Kurtis, most of my symptoms had subsided, and all we could go on were my accounts of what was happening that spring and summer and my current symptomology. "Your brain wants to heal. We see a lot of this stuff happen when people get off these types of medications." He was the first doctor to really understand that this existed. What a relief to know that I wasn't going crazy! I wanted to break down and cry. I wanted to hug this man.

Why didn't I bring Scott? I thought. *He needs to hear this.*

"What do I do about the medication I'm on now?" I asked, wanting to spend the whole afternoon with him now that I knew he was competent. "You may just have to stay on this medication for now. We can probably slowly remove it as your brain heals more." We agreed to monitor the situation and meet as needed.

There were no treatment options that I hadn't already tried for this, other than a blood pressure pill, which he advised against based on my current symptomology. There was a new drug on the market called tetrabenazine, which just seemed to make people more depressed rather than helping with controlling movements. He advised against that as well.

In my car, I smiled as I cried tears of joy. My mind had so much information in it I wanted to explode. I wanted to call everyone to tell them that finally I had found someone who could help.

So that was it. Stay the course on the meds, monitor, and, over time, slowly remove the meds. That made sense. I had a plan. I felt like I had gotten my life back in Dr. Kurtis' office. Even though I wasn't one hundred percent functioning, he was right. Time seemed to be helping me, and I felt good at the prospect of someday getting off these meds. While I didn't fully agree with the speculative tardive dyskinesia diagnosis, because my symptoms seemed a little more complex than that, at least he was the first doctor who was aware that such things could happen from these types of medications.

I felt that a weight had been lifted off my shoulders and that I could move forward and try again. Genuine hope had been restored.

After that, everyone was pushing me to get back to life. "An idle mind is the Devil's playground," Dr. Lewis would say, knowing that I was still hesitant to go back to work.

A few weeks later, in March 2013, I cautiously returned to work, slowly inching back into my old life. I made sure my client load would be light—I was only going to be there one day a week. Walking in on that first day I was incredibly nervous. My colleagues greeted me like the psychiatric patient I was. "Are you feeling okay? Are you sure you're up for this?" they asked in soft voices.

With each passing day, the movements would settle. My body was coming back to me. That spring I resubmitted all of the necessary paperwork to go off to school in the fall. I had been so worried that I had given up my chance, but I got in . . . again. It wasn't as exciting as the first time, but what counted most was that they reaccepted me. My body still wasn't perfect, but I was able to take things one day at a time with a new sense of hope.

It would be several years before I could truly feel leveled out. Edmund became known as my "movement disorder" to Scott and my friends. He started to fade into the background as his power grew weaker over me. I was able to live life without him consuming my waking hours. The medicine I was taking was working. I went on with my life as best as I could. There were days I would even forget that Edmund was a part of me.

My next goal was to get off the remaining medication. That's when I would truly be free of this past part of myself, free to live without the worries of this thing haunting me. But Edmund was not done with me yet. He still had a third act to perform.

PART III

"The Wheele is come full circle; I am heere."
— William Shakespeare
King Lear, Edmund (Bastard), Act 5, Scene 3, line 3136
(*First Folio Edition, Folio I* 1623)

CHAPTER 28
Graduate School

My first class the day I walked into the Lincoln Center Campus of Fordham University was Human Rights and Social Justice. I took a seat in the back, trying not to be noticed. This felt like a *real* university, not the performing arts school I had gone to back in college, and I was incredibly anxious that morning.

"I assume you all read the article for today," the professor said as the final arrivals took their seats.

Some students nodded at him, but there were plenty of us who looked at each other puzzled and terrified as if we had committed a crime.

"You're graduate students, not children. Look at the syllabus," he told us.

All of my classes were packed into one day to leave time for my internship on the remaining days of the week. After sitting through a full day of classes and having my mind filled with information about what was expected of me this semester, I was shaken. My mind was trying to figure out how I was going to do all this work.

Scott picked me up after that first long day and treated me to dinner with his friend Tiff. We walked across the street and down a block to an overpriced shitty diner that masqueraded as a high-end restaurant.

"So, tell me! How was your first day?" Scott asked excitedly as he took the bag full of encyclopedia-sized books off my shoulder. Lost in thought of all the homework I had that first night, I said, "Um, this is like *real* school. I'm already late on some of my homework."

Scott smiled and chuckled. "You're going to be fine." He was way more excited than I was about this experience. I was just glad I made it through the day without Edmund making an appearance.

Scott joked, "Now you get to make some money when this is all done."

It didn't take me long to realize that I made the right decision. Yes, the work was hard, but after the first semester, I was falling in love with my new career. Getting to understand the dynamics of human behavior and development, social policy, and how to work with patients was rewarding personally and professionally. In addition, as an actor/writer/painter, it gave me so much material about the human experience.

During my first year I interned at a hospital/nursing home. I worked with elderly individuals who either had no money or who had been abandoned by their families and were now basically property of the state. Side note: If your children hate you or you think that you won't be able to depend on your children in your old age, get long-term care insurance. You don't want to end up at one of these places. The facility always smelled like feces and unshowered bodies. The lack of care from staff was horrifying.

At this internship I made a new friend, Yuliya, a Slovakian woman who was also returning to school later in life. We commiserated over our field placement and shared our appalling experiences of working at the state-run nursing home. Once, we tried to start a campaign to get the residents, as they were known, more fruit in their diet, a true delicacy in a place that offered nothing more than processed food. Our efforts did not end well, and we were told to stop "riling up the residents."

At school we had a professor who whipped us into shape if we handed in a paper with poor grammar or if it didn't meet APA requirements.

Even though she was a stickler for formatting, she also taught us how to be great social workers and would become one of my favorite teachers.

Yuliya and I connected instantly on our ideologies and life experiences. We also both had ambitions of one day starting our own private practices. Our field advisor was a kind, elderly woman, who was literally working her way to the grave. She even had a heart attack one day at our field placement. Luckily, she survived. We selfish interns had been worried that we wouldn't get credit if she died. Yuliya and I made a pact that if either one of us went down at this hospital, we would drive the other to a better facility.

What made our supervisor so special was that she wanted us to find our place within the field. She encouraged us to visit other facilities where we might want to do our next internship. "You can visit a hospital, homeless shelter, or even a correctional facility," she said at one of our weekly meetings.

Correctional facility? There was something fascinating about that. I had watched plenty of TV shows about the lives of individuals behind bars. I wondered how you would work with them. I made sure we visited a local county jail. Wow, this was not just any jail. During our tour, Yuliya commented, "I can't believe the jail is cleaner than the nursing home."

While it was definitely a jail, what made the place so impressive was that they had entire clinical programs serving all parts of the population. This jail had an entire drug and alcohol rehab facility located within the concrete walls. I met two of the social workers that day and got to hear what a day looked like for them.

I loved the thought of challenging myself, and my heart instantly went out to these incarcerated individuals who didn't have many people advocating for them. It felt like a great place to make a real difference. After visiting that jail, it didn't take me long to decide where I wanted to do my next internship. I persistently nudged the social worker in charge of interns and had my field advisor pester her as well. Finally, I got an interview and ultimately got in there for my next field placement.

This was one of the greatest experiences of my life. I loved getting to work with people who seemed to actually need help, and I loved all of the programs that they were running.

They asked me to start an art group, which turned out to be a valuable learning experience for me but started out on a sour note.

"Ladies, we need to collect the crayons and make sure they're all accounted for after each group. Two of them are missing," I said to the women as I clapped my hands like I was talking to school children.

Parodying the pitch of my voice, one of them said, "You must have miscounted." Other hecklers laughed and agreed. Enraged, I went off the wall, raising my voice, screaming at them, hoping to get one of them to fess up. This only encouraged more laughter as they manipulated the situation and turned it around on me.

"It's not our fault you lost them," one said.

Another said, "You didn't even bring a full pack in with you."

No one came forward. I was furious. Later, when I talked to a lieutenant about the incident, I found out that one of the ladies had in fact taken the missing crayons.

"Why would they steal the crayons?" I asked the lieutenant as I sat in his office, dumbfounded that they would destroy my group and terrified that I would be let go from this internship because of my carelessness in not collecting all the crayons.

He laughed at my naiveté. "They use them for makeup."

"For who?"

Amused at my amazement, he said, "They try to flirt with the guys as they pass them in the hallways."

"Huh . . . and where did they hide them?" I asked, genuinely curious about where these crayons could be hidden with such little privacy. I caught myself when I realized what a stupid question that was. He confirmed my suspicions. "They hid them in their privates. When you guys left, they tried flushing them down the toilet, but they ended up flooding the unit . . ."

Poetic justice, I thought.

The lieutenant reassured me, "Don't feel bad, I would have yelled at them too."

It wasn't my proudest moment as a social worker. But what I loved about the jail was that it was a place where I could learn from exceptional clinicians, who helped me develop bona fide clinical skills as a social worker. My supervisor had me turn the experience into a "clinical moment," and my next session with the group was devoted to processing why they stole the crayons and what this meant on a deeper level.

There was a position opening up at the jail when I graduated, but my inability to speak Spanish put me out of the running. I wasn't even considered, but over the years I kept in touch with my supervisor.

Graduating with my master's was one of the greatest achievements of my life. Our ceremony was at Lincoln Center, which felt like a full-circle moment from my acting days. I always wanted to be on one of their stages, and here I was. My dad came up to New York to see me walk down the aisle and get my diploma on that stage. Mom was not there, of course.

Shortly after graduation would be the last time I ever spoke with my mother. I couldn't take the hot and cold relationship anymore, and every time we did speak it felt like I was walking on eggshells. As a child, I didn't have the knowledge or language to understand what was wrong with my mother, but since going to graduate school, I learned that there was a disorder whose description seemed to fit her. I know as clinicians we're not supposed to diagnose friends and family (and that is not what I am doing here), but her symptomology seemed to fit the bill for borderline personality disorder. And, as I looked back at my entire life with her, it made perfect sense. BPD, as it is often known, is a condition in which a person struggles to manage their emotions, amongst other things. It's a hard disorder to understand, and there are a lot of components to it, but one of the key features is trouble with interpersonal relationships. My mother always struggled with this.

As a graduation present, Scott took me to a spa weekend in Montreal. His intentions were very sweet, but I always hated other massage therapists working on me, because many were so poorly trained. Nevertheless, it was the thought that counted, and I let go of my preconceived ideas, and we drove to Canada the summer after graduation.

We were driving down the highway, right before we hit the Canadian border, when my phone rang. Looking at the caller ID, I could see that it was my mother. I showed it to Scott, who begged me, "Please don't answer it." I answered anyway, hoping that I could make it a quick conversation.

The minute I answered, she started dumping her problems on me. It was something about how she was trying to get into some special housing for lower-income individuals. From the panicked and angry tone in her voice, I could sense that my mother was nervous knowing that her funds would soon be depleted with my dad's alimony checks coming to an end within a few months.

Now that I was a social worker, I tried to ease her worries. "I can help you with assisted living and housing when I get back, if you want. I know some of the ins-and-outs of that." Her tone got angrier and she became belligerent. "You think you're so fancy now that you're a doctor, you think you can help me. I don't need your help."

I wasn't a doctor, I was a master level clinician, but that was beside the point. A switch turned on in me during her tirade. I was offering to help, and as she did so many times in the past, she turned the situation around and berated me. The years of repressed anger and frustration I felt toward this woman couldn't be held in any longer. It was as if an entire lifetime of hurt came pouring out of me. I screamed louder than I've ever screamed at anyone. "You miserable, selfish woman!" I laid into her about how mean she was and that she made everyone's life a living hell.

"This will absolutely be the last time you and I ever communicate. I never want to hear from you again." I paused and waited for her response.

"Hello?"

She had hung up on me. Those were the last words I ever said to her.

I had a visceral reaction and wailed out a guttural scream as I sat there in the car with Scott.

In an attempt to console me, he was rubbing my back with the one arm that he wasn't using to drive. "Oh, honey, I'm sorry."

That was it. I had never done anything wrong to this woman. I had always tried my best with her. Even though it felt uneasy and unsettling to make this decision, I vowed that we would part ways and that I would never see her again. I would never again answer the phone if she called; never again open another letter from her. In that moment she died, and I wouldn't shed one more tear for her. We could never coexist in the same space.

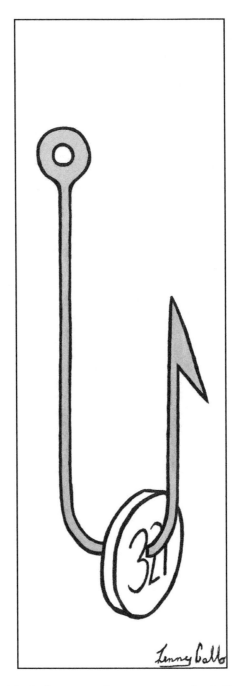

Hooked, 2013, oil on canvas, 12" x 36".

CHAPTER 29

Hooked

During my entire time in school and after, Edmund never really went away. He was always there, but never with the same intensity as when it began. During periods of stress and high pressure, I had "episodes" where my body became restless, and I couldn't sit still. Sometimes it would be nothing more than a day, while other times it could go on for a week. It was nothing I couldn't manage, nothing more than a few movements here and there.

One thing I could not let go of during my time at Fordham and after graduating was that I was still on the remaining medication. Dr. Kurtis' words of tapering over time resonated with me, and I was determined to do this, and felt that, with just enough time, I would gradually be able to get off all pills. Originally, Dr. Lewis was on board with this plan as well.

Early on, before I started school, Dr. Lewis and I would try to lower doses of the meds slowly. I got to some very low points in the process, as much as half the medicine could be out of my system, but there would always come a point when I got too low, and the movements would return stronger. In a panic, I would call him, and to solve the problem, we would just go back up on the meds. They never came back with the same intensity, but it would take months to reregulate my body.

Dr. Lewis saw what happened to me every time I lowered my meds. He saw my disappointment and how this wasn't giving me a decent quality of life. Often, he said to me in a somber tone, "Len, I think we're going to have to accept that this is probably as good as it's going to get." Hearing that felt like a knife in the chest. I struggled to accept this reality. I didn't want this to be the way it ended. Why couldn't I get off these pills? Dr. Lewis really believed that if it's not broken, don't fix it.

Dr. Kurtis, on the other hand, thought that I was still young enough to give it a try and see if I could get off all the remaining meds. He suggested giving it time, and later, trying again. Regardless of what either of them thought, I wanted off these pills. There was a time in my life when I wasn't hooked on these things, and I wanted to get back to that time. At this point I was left with 1.5mg of Ativan, 37.5 milligrams of Benadryl, and 600 milligrams of Trileptal.

From time to time, I tapered the pills on my own without telling either one of them. I tried tapering through Fordham, breaking my promise to Dr. Lewis that I wouldn't taper during school. When I graduated, I tried then, too. I tried all through my first job at a drug rehab facility, where, ironically, I was helping other people who were trying to get off substances themselves.

Each time my condition worsened, I called Dr. Lewis, crying, and we started to go back to my original dose. He never said it, but I could always hear his voice through his sad, frustrated smile: "Stop fucking with your meds, just stay on the pills and move on with your life."

Fuck that. I knew how addictive benzodiazepines could be and did not want to be on these pills and have them control the rest of my life. And just what were they doing inside my head? Were they still helping my disorder? I also feared that one day I would become dependent on these pills, or maybe I already was. There was enough data out there suggesting that these pills should only be used for short periods of time and that I should get off the medications. Every time I tried, I ended up causing myself weeks to months of movements. Feelings of defeat consumed my mind. How the hell was I going to get off these things?

In July 2016, I got a text from my former supervisor at the jail. "There's an opening, and I'm telling them to hire you." I was ecstatic. A government job, pension, good health insurance, and a chance to run the drug program? This was the opportunity I had been waiting for. The hiring process was lengthy. It consisted of a background check that basically started at the day I was born. They wanted documents from places that no longer existed from when I was a teenager.

Once I was hired at the jail, I thought I would stay there for at least most of my career. I got to take back my art group, which was still running. My boss was incredibly flexible and allowed me to try pretty much anything I wanted. I got to start an LGBTQ+ group for immigrant detainees; I got to bring a lot of fun ideas into the drug program; and I even was able to get supplies that were deemed contraband into the place. Some of my writing about my experiences got published in trade magazines. But, as anyone in the work world knows, sometimes management and policies change and new rules are set. The things that initially brought me to the jail were slowly fading away, and within a very short time, the jail turned into something way different from what it had been.

In addition to the changing structure, my boss was leaving. Also, I wasn't getting paid enough, and my attempts to get a raise were ignored by people in higher positions than my boss. When I came from working in the drug rehab facility to the jail, it was a lateral move. I didn't get into social work expecting to be rich, but I didn't think that it was right to have a master's degree without a little more pay. I was still working part-time at my massage job to supplement my salary.

It had been a while since my friend Yuliya and I had talked, and I called to see how she was doing. I learned that she was in the process of starting her private practice.

"Where are you seeing your clients?" I asked, trying to figure out how she was doing a private practice without an office.

"In my house." *Is she mad? Is she trying to get killed?* Having worked in the jail and drug rehab facility, I forgot that not everyone who was seeking therapy had been accused of a crime and was trying to manipulate you. Everyday people went to therapy as well.

"Is that legal?"

"Yes, it is. A lot of therapists have home practices." The wheels in my brain started spinning, and excitedly I went into problem-solving mode. She wasn't wrong. There were groups and online forums on how to start a therapy practice from home. Was this something I could do? I couldn't stop thinking about why I was not taking her lead.

"Scott and I have a separate part of our house that might make for a good office," I told Yuliya.

"Give it a shot. You could always do part-time and see," she suggested.

"How many patients do you have?" I asked, still trying to comprehend that she was actually going for something that we had merely talked about in grad school.

"Twelve." I did the math in my head, and my eyes lit up with the possibilities of what could be.

Our conversation sparked a new bit of inspiration in me. I could give up my massage job and make up the difference. I could also start to establish my practice so that in five years, when my loans were forgiven, I could leave the jail and eventually do a full-time private practice. I wouldn't have to rent an office space right away. Having my own practice had always been my goal, and here was an opportunity to do that.

I had long talks with Scott, researched everything I could, and consulted with Yuliya weekly. By November 2018, I was ready to take on my first patient.

All was going well, and I was making positive changes. Running, something I never thought I would do, became a routine part of my days, and I was preparing to train for a marathon. Scott and I traveled when we could. I was eating healthier, losing weight, and finding some balance in my life.

Each year the *Dystonia Medical Research Foundation* had an event to raise money and awareness. Gene, the woman who guided me at that meeting years ago, was the coordinator of this event. I was always grateful to Gene for telling me about movement disorder specialists, and now that I was a social worker I was able to give back. Many of these individuals were still struggling. At the very least, I wanted to help support them with the hope of helping them out of their nightmare, because it looked like I was out of mine.

Normally, I had a yearly follow-up with Dr. Kurtis, but it had been a few years since I had seen him. I was feeling good enough, and there really wasn't a need. I actually started referring patients with neurological disorders to him and thought of him more as a colleague now. Dr. Lewis and I seemed to be managing just fine with what we were doing.

Then came COVID.

CHAPTER 30
"What Have I Done?"

As COVID plagued the nation in the spring of 2020, my private practice, which was relatively new, turned into a virtual practice. Nobody knew what this thing was or how it was going to affect their lives, and everyone was worried that they were going to catch this disease.

When you work at a jail, you catch everything, so I figured it was only a matter of time before I got it. COVID spread throughout the jail like wildfire. Mental health was deemed essential, which meant we had no choice; we went to work and prayed that it didn't kill us.

Everyone was stuck at home binge-watching TV, wiping their groceries down with bleach and other cleaning products, and struggling to find toilet paper. But in all this madness there were pockets of hope and changes all across the country in positive ways. People were working from home and spending more time with their families. Everyone was reassessing their values, something I got to see firsthand in my virtual private practice patients. They were making major life decisions, questioning what they wanted to do for work moving forward and if they ever wanted to return to an office. They were deciding if they could spend the rest of their lives with their spouses and whether or not they wanted children. The world was changing rapidly.

The jail finally decided that on-duty staff would be pared down to a minimum in an attempt to lower the spread of COVID. This meant one person from mental health always had to be working at the jail. Wanting to capitalize on as much free time off as we could get, one of my colleagues and I agreed to split the weeks. Sometimes we each, in turn, got as much as eight days off. This enabled me to reassess my own values and gave me a much-needed break to think about what I was doing.

I realized that as much as I loved being a social worker, I was sick of working for people. I'm not a team player, I'll own that. I'm too much of an independent thinker to work under others, and I don't like to sit through meetings that could have been emails. I don't like following the rules. I like to think outside the box, and I don't like to be micromanaged. I'm not a good employee, and this became quite evident while working in an institution with as much structure as the jail.

My social work career was supposed to offer the balance that would allow me to do art and theatre, but I was burning out. I missed my art and my writing. It was getting harder to go into the jail and keep from criticizing all the changes that were taking place. The drug program I ran had shut down due to COVID. The new people in charge started to change the dynamic of the institution, and I was becoming very unhappy.

Yuliya and I talked weekly, and she kept encouraging me to give a full-time therapy practice a shot. "You don't need an office to do this. You can build up your caseload without having to put the money out," she told me.

I started going through all the numbers and scenarios in my head, but I couldn't bring myself to take the plunge. Fear and anxiety still dominated parts of my life. I had a good job with great health insurance. Did I really want to give that up? Plus, I was working toward loan forgiveness on a program that required me to work in the public sector for ten years. After that, any remaining balance on my loan would be forgiven. If I gave up the jail, I would be responsible for paying back the full amount of the loan.

The idea of tapering off the pills once again entered my mind. I'm not sure why, but I felt that this might be a good time to do it. My running put me in some of the best shape I'd ever been. Maybe I was bored during COVID. Some might argue that it was self-sabotaging, but as I reflected on my life thus far, it seemed that using the pills was the one thing that was holding me back. And every time I had to take one, I was reminded that Edmund was still present in my life—I hated that. The idea that I was still on those pills and was giving money to the drug companies bothered me greatly.

The last time I tried tapering was when I was at the drug rehab facility where I worked. It had been so long since I had tried to get off these pills, I wondered if I needed them anymore. Maybe I could do this now, I thought.

I didn't dare bring this up with Dr. Lewis, who I assumed would most likely discourage me from making this decision. I figured I could certainly cut back the dosages a little on my own and see what happened. I had done it before. If anything happened, I would just go back up as we had in the past. This was a test, I told myself. If I had any excess agitation that was being caused by the taper, it could easily be handled if I just ran it off.

For this round of tapering, I decided to start with a quarter of my Ativan in the afternoon dose. I broke the pill into four pieces and took three of the pieces.

Nothing happened, nothing negative at all that first day.

A week went by, nothing.

Two more weeks passed, and still nothing. I wasn't feeling worse. My agitation levels were low. Edmund was in check.

I was excited. I'd reached this point on previous tapers. Could I actually cross the finish line this time?

When a month had passed with no problems, I decided to lower my dose by another quarter.

Still nothing.

Maybe my body really was ready to get off these things.

In late June of that year, something didn't feel quite right. I was now down a full pill. I was getting a terrible case of tinnitus that wasn't going away. Being the fitness queen that I now was, I paid attention to my Apple watch, which informed me that I was getting less and less sleep each night as well. Then came the anxiety, followed by migraines. I figured that my body would just need time to settle and that the tapering of the medication was doing its thing. After all, I concluded, nothing horrible was happening, and, once again, I figured this wasn't anything I couldn't handle.

On the morning of July 16, I woke up after getting only four hours of sleep. It was my week to work, and I had one day left before my colleague started doing her days. As I made my morning coffee, I began to shake and feel bolts of energy flashing through me. I thought: *NO, THIS IS NOT WHAT I THINK IT IS . . . is it?*

My movements were wilder than they had been in a very long time. This wasn't the usual little hiccup; this was a bit more intense. Hoping that this was a fluke, I brushed it off and got ready for work. *I can handle this*, I told myself, figuring that I was just going to be a little extra squirmy that day. As I drove to work, I tried deep breathing to calm myself, but my mind wouldn't stop racing.

No, this isn't happening. Is it? Edmund is that you? No part of me wanted to believe that I had brought this thing back into my life.

As I did in prior years, I walked into work and did my best to keep it together. But now I wouldn't have my little massage room to crawl off into. I had to assess people's mental health and make the appropriate referrals for them. I had to walk into jail cells with people who were having psychotic breakdowns, while trying to work through these movements. I struggled to sit at my desk. I struggled to write my notes. All the while, my mind told me: *Breathe. Just keep it together. You can get through this.*

I don't remember what it was, but the day before I had made a decision that one of my colleagues disagreed with. Now I was being

211

called into my new boss's office. My Apple watch indicated that my resting heart rate was at one hundred and fifty beats per minute. My thoughts were racing, and my body was starting to panic. I struggled to listen as my colleague screamed at me in front of my new boss. I can't tell you most of what my colleague said, but I remember hearing the words "incompetent" and "negligence." I kept repeating to myself: *Calm down. Almost 4:00 p.m. When you get home, you will go back to the regular doses of medicine, and this will start to settle. You're almost at the end of the day.*

I realized that clearly this test was failing, and I would have to cut my losses and go back to the doses I had been on.

When my shift ended, I rushed to my car and drove home. As soon as I got inside, I took the prescribed doses of the pills—but it was too late. The feeling of terror that had remained dormant for nearly eight years had come back. I never thought I would experience that again. Edmund had been rebirthed.

Oh, God, what have I done?

Agitation consumed me. Much like the first time, I couldn't tell you what I was afraid of, but I was filled with an overall, abstract terror. Edmund *never* came back with this intensity in my previous tapers, but here he was. Did I destroy my life? I begged God to give me a chance to redeem myself.

"Scott! The terror and paranoia! I can't get it under control."

He looked at me, somewhat confused. "What?"

I repeated myself, but he knew what I meant. He rubbed my back and told me that everything was going to be okay, but the look of horror in his eyes said something different. He knew that I had unleashed Edmund.

"Call Dr. Lewis," Scott said.

I was already thinking the same thing. I had to fess up, and I called him in a rush of panic. He was with patients, so I told his front desk staff to ask him to contact me before he left for the day and that it was an emergency.

When Dr. Lewis called, he sounded surprised to hear from me. "What's going on? I just saw you a month ago."

"I fucked up," I admitted, tears running down my face like a child who knew he had done wrong.

"What?" he said.

"I fucked up. I started tapering again. It's back."

It seemed like an eternity of silence on the other end of the phone. By the sound of his breathing, I could tell he was upset. As calmly as he could, Dr. Lewis said, "Okay. Let's figure this out. We have to put it back in the box."

Yes, I thought. *Please, let's figure this out quickly.* I had so much respect for Dr. Lewis, I felt terrible having to tell him what I had done.

I called my new boss and my colleagues to let them know that I was having a medical emergency and would keep them posted.

That week, Dr. Lewis and I tried to level out my medications. I thought we would just raise the doses, and in a few days—or weeks at most, this would work itself out. That wasn't happening. Every time we went up, my symptoms got worse. It was as if the medication that had been controlling things for so many years had turned on me. I was in such disbelief I didn't even know how to feel about this. But the ambiguous terror and movements were back and dominated my thoughts.

Dr. Lewis encouraged me to schedule an appointment with Dr. Kurtis. I was way ahead of him and had called a few days prior. Now that I wasn't one of his regular patients anymore, the soonest I would be able to get in with Dr. Kurtis would be a month. During this month, Dr. Lewis and I tried as best as we could try to level out my meds, but nothing seemed to be working.

Once again in my life I had to call my boss and say I was going to be out for an undetermined amount of time. Once again I had to figure out the finances. And once again I had to let go of something that I had been working toward for a long time.

"I need to refer you to another therapist," I told my private patients, letting them know I would be on medical leave for a while.

Edmund was back. There was no denying it.

In a last-ditch effort to try and level me out, I begged Dr. Lewis to put me on another medication. I had known since my early days of having this disorder that a blood pressure pill by the name of Propranolol was considered a treatment option for medication-induced movement disorders. He agreed, and that afternoon I took half of the lowest dose of that pill. It enabled me to settle a bit, but the minute the pill wore off, my symptoms were even worse. By day three, the pill wasn't helping at all. I would have to wait for my appointment with Dr. Kurtis.

CHAPTER 31

"You've Got Everything."

Back in 2012, when this first happened to me, there was very little literature that I could find online about medication-induced movement disorders. But by 2020, there was a lot more on the subject, which included Facebook groups dedicated to those afflicted by them. I joined every one of these groups. To my surprise, as I scrolled through, I found that everyone was talking about similar symptoms: the inability to stop moving, as well as myriad other issues, including the terror they were experiencing. I also learned something that was even harder to digest: people were getting this from benzodiazepines as well.

While there was now a lot of research on movement disorders related to antipsychotics, there was very little on withdrawing from benzos. Most of the research seemed to be predominantly focused on antipsychotics. So, if going down on a benzo made it worse and going up on a benzo made it worse, then what were my options? Did I even have any?

Scott drove me to Dr. Kurtis' office. I sat there moving in the car, trying not to let the terror overtake my body. He rubbed my back and stayed calm the entire drive. Several years earlier he had started an intensive practice in Martial Arts and Tai Chi, which gave him a stillness that emanated from all aspects of his personality. The whole process felt very surreal, like we were living in a loop of a past version of ourselves. I felt so guilty for putting him through this again. My body was curling and I was crying. Scott remained silent.

Dr. Kurtis had a new office in West Milford, New Jersey. While telehealth and telemedicine were now the preferred options for meeting since COVID, he wanted to see me in person for the first visit. We entered his office with our masks on. He was now in a much quainter space than the hospital he used to work at. He smiled when he came out to greet us, but as soon as he saw the state I was in, that smile turned to a more serious and sadder look. "It's been a while," he uttered.

Tears streaming from my eyes, I looked at him hopelessly. He took Scott and me into his office, where he began his assessment and tried to gather information.

"How did this start?" he asked, while jostling my legs.

I turned to see Scott, who was sitting across from me, staring in my direction. Then Dr. Kurtis made eye contact with me, and the words spewed from my mouth. "I lowered my Ativan. I was fine at first, but as soon as I noticed the movements come back, we went back up and that started making things worse. Nothing we were doing was leveling this out. Dr. Lewis and I tried Propranolol."

"That would have been my first choice for this," he said as he checked my eyes.

I'm glad you're on the same page.

Confused and trying to gauge his facial expressions, I asked, "What is going on with me?"

He was still trying to assess: "Pull down your mask and open your mouth."

I obliged and held my breath so as not to release my acrid smoker's breath into his face. He saw how I couldn't hold my jaw still: it was going side to side. He observed the movements the rest of my body was making.

In that moment, he saw the full range of what Edmund looked like in action and what had happened to me years prior when I got off Geodon and Risperdal. I was not expecting his next words. He looked me dead in the eye, took hold of my shoulders, and said, "You've got everything."

What did he mean by everything? My mind started to connect the dots.

"So, this is tardive akathisia?" I asked, trying to get a confirmation. Without a pause he said, "Yes."

"And tardive dyskinesia?"

"Yes. Everything. You've even got Tourette's."

My mind was still trying to process the word *everything*, and I attempted to focus and further clarify what he had just said: "Because of the medication?"

"Yes, this is all because of the medication."

I asked him about the terror I was feeling. "Your brain is trying to level out, and there's a lot of cross-firing going on. It's more of a withdrawal-induced paranoia. You're not going crazy. It's all connected. You have tardive syndrome."

If I wasn't moving so much and my body wasn't squirming all over the place, I would have hugged him. Finally, I had a diagnosis. It was the restlessness of akathisia. It was the jerky movements of tardive dyski-nesia. And to top it off, I had tic-like movements in a medication-in-duced form of Tourette's, along with some withdrawal-induced paranoia just for shits and giggles. The wrath that Edmund had set loose on me had been named, and it all made sense in that moment.

The unexplained terror, the constant movements, the ups and downs on medications, all the pieces in this puzzle started to fall into place. My terror at seeing the taillights on the Mercedes as I drove down Ridge Road that Mother's Day after cutting out the Geodon; the inability to sit still and incessant pacing before I was committed to the psych ward at St. Dominic's after my taper from Risperdal—in this moment it all came together. This is what I had; there was no more guessing. In his ten-minute assessment, Dr. Kurtis had officially diagnosed me and given me answers I thought I would never get.

He went with tardive syndrome because no one movement super-seded the other, although the akathisia and tics were the most prevalent when I saw Dr. Kurtis that day. This was all brought about by the use of Reglan and psychiatric medications, and this latest round because of a fast taper of the benzodiazepines.

Relieved that I was right, my mind turned back to the problem that confronted us. Trying to keep my composure, I asked, "So, what do we do about this?"

Dr. Kurtis was optimistic. "There's stuff we can do. Treatment has come a long way since you first had this, but mostly it will require more time and waiting."

Initially, Dr. Kurtis wanted to put me on the newest treatment for tardive dyskinesia: VMAT II inhibitors. These medicines were promising for tardive dyskinesia and now were even being advertised on TV. The cost of this regimen started at about sixty thousand dollars a year, and no insurance would cover it. Dr. Kurtis believed they would work for everything I had going on. He told me about other patients with similar issues, who had tried them with success. But there was a drawback: possible side effects.

He handed me a brochure for the newest one of these pills. My fingers opened the glossy pamphlet, and my eyes quickly, almost reflexively, went to the fine print. Side effects may include drooling. *I could handle that.* Falling asleep randomly. *Please give me that one.* And may cause akathisia. *Hold the horses.*

What amazed me about the new VMAT II inhibitors was that they could help or cause and worsen movement disorders. How does something help and have the potential for hurting at the same time? This was the same shit with the psychiatric meds, which could cause paradoxical symptoms and do the opposite of what they were supposed to do for you. I did not want to take the risk.

"So, this could make the akathisia worse?"

"It could," Dr. Kurtis said, "but I don't think that will happen."

I never thought I'd be in a position to know what the word akathisia meant; yet here we are!

"What are my other options?" I asked, rejecting that pill immediately.

"We can put you on Amantadine."

"I've tried that before. It made me nauseous."

"Perhaps the dose was too high. We have to try something. Maybe you just take one pill at bedtime. We need to calm down your receptors. That's the goal here right now."

My brain was always jumping ten miles down the road, and I didn't know what to do. I looked at Scott. He didn't seem to know what to say. This was up to me to decide. Ever since this happened, I was terrified of medicine. I could barely take an aspirin. My body had gotten some of the rarer side effects from pills. Did I want to chance it again? But did I really have a choice? I was so scared, I couldn't make a rational decision.

Dr. Kurtis saw my torment. "How about we start you on Amantadine and just see? You can always take the other pill." I knew it would make me nauseous, but if it could just get me out of this terror state and enable me to get some sleep, I would gladly vomit at this point. That was really my only option: take the medicine and begin the waiting game.

"Fine, let's do Amantadine," I told him.

"Okay. And we'll leave the Ativan at the dose you were at before you tapered, and you won't change that for now."

All this, only to wind up right back where I started.

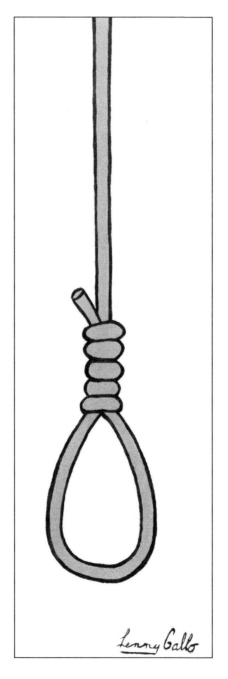

Suicide Awareness, 2020, oil on canvas, 10" x 30".

CHAPTER 32

Death

I thought about doing more paintings, but I couldn't find the motivation. I couldn't do my running, my practice was gone, and now Edmund would once again control my life. Waiting and time; that was all I could do. I felt paralyzed with fear and wondered daily if my decision to taper had simply given Edmund full control and permanent reign over my life. I couldn't find the mental clarity to put anything together, with the exception of one piece that I painted on a long, thin, ten-by-thirty canvas, one of my favorite sizes.

When the symptoms recurred the second time, I'd be lying if I said that taking my life wasn't a constant theme that I had to stave off. Having this happen once seemed like a lesson to learn; twice felt like a cruel joke. It's hard to talk about this, because I considered myself a Renaissance Man. I wanted to experience everything this earth had to offer. Take my life? Please, who has time for that? Who would want to do such a thing when there are so many opportunities in life?

I found that to survive this disorder in its most acute phases, I had to be willing to let go of everything. All I thought I knew about time went out the window. I had no control over anything in my body. I never knew how I was going to feel from one moment to the next, and

I had no choice but to try to be as fully present in each moment as possible . . . and wait.

Creeping in was that all-too-familiar feeling. The sensation of emptiness that I had felt years ago penetrated my soul once again. Edmund had taken so much from me; I didn't want to let him take any more.

You can't just go around telling people that you want to kill yourself, because you'd wind up getting committed, and I had already been down that road. The truth is that when you are in the midst of this torment, death feels like a relief. I didn't spend much time thinking about how my death might impact Scott or my dad and friends. Just imagine for a moment the continuous torture of moving, agitation, and uncertainty, versus the eternal restfulness of sleep that one supposes death would bring. I began to welcome death with open arms and prayed that God would do me the favor of taking my life so as not to have to commit the act myself.

Many people have taken their lives from medication-induced movement disorders. A point comes when the human body can only take so much and doesn't want to fight anymore. Let me be very clear. I didn't want to die. What I wanted was relief from the torture. I wanted my life back. But you don't get that very quickly with this disorder. I didn't dare share my thoughts with anyone. I believe that my social work training helped keep me alive. Once, I went to a training on suicide ideation. The instructor said something that hit home and changed my thoughts on the subject: "We're never going to stop people from killing themselves; those who have thoughts of self-harm rarely share them with others. If you encounter one of the few people who is serious about wanting to take their life *and* who is brave enough to share it with you, don't frighten them off. Don't try and get them to see the light. Don't tell them everything will be all right. Just validate them and remind them that they can have those thoughts all they want . . . they just don't have to take any action today."

UNSTILL

That was the narrative that ran through my mind every day. *You don't have to do this today . . . you don't have to do this today.* On some level I knew that I hadn't explored all my options, and I vowed to myself that I would not go down this permanent road without exhausting every last opportunity, even if death felt for now like the best solution.

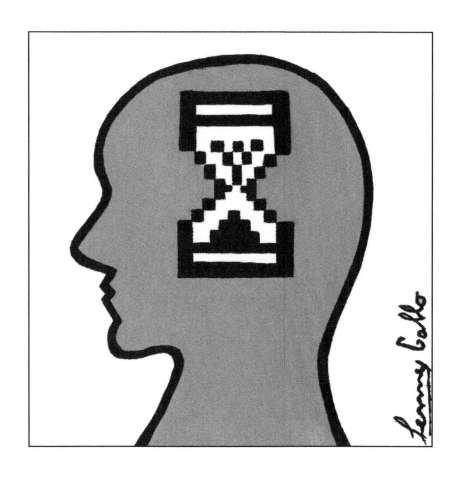

Waiting, Part II, 2012, oil on canvas, 10" x 10".

CHAPTER 33
Waiting Part II

That summer went by much as the first summer had. My old routine came right back. The only difference this time was that we were also dealing with an infestation of yellow jackets that buzzed every morning as they flew through the air conditioning vents of our house. Those fuckers were a bitch to get rid of, but it gave me something to focus on.

Dr. Lewis and I were back to meeting every other week so I could fill him in on my progress. During one of the sessions, which were now held by videoconference, I asked, "What do you think is wrong with me?"

"What do you mean?" he asked, unsure of what I was looking for him to say.

"This can't all be anxiety. Why do you think I'm like this?"

He went silent. Whenever I asked him a question that he didn't want to answer he would stare at me for a few moments. I could tell he was trying to choose his words carefully. He said gently, "You probably have a mild case of OCD as well."

Bullshit, I thought. I've worked with people with OCD, and I don't have any of the rituals that are a distinguishing part of OCD. But I had to respect his theory. "Maybe," I told him, not one hundred percent convinced.

225

Also, Dr. Kurtis and I were meeting every other week to check on my progress.

During one of my appointments, Dr. Kurtis explained the condition to me like this: "Your brain has a forest fire going on inside of it. We can try to use medicines to help you go through the fire more easily, but, in the end, the fire must burn out . . . and time is the only thing that can make that happen."

So, I waited, and I waited again, as I had before. I binge-watched TV seasons. I watched the entire series of *Lucifer*. Finally, I found out what all the *Game of Thrones* hype was about. Nick and I were back to our daily conversations, although this time the tone was more somber. Scott once again took care of meals and rubbed my legs and arms at night to try and keep me calm. Yuliya and other friends checked in on me weekly.

My sick time would run out in September, and fears of money once again surfaced. I was approaching forty, and my expenses were much higher than when this originally started, yet all I could do was wait for my brain to level out enough for me to be able to function.

Time was a word that I came to dread, but it seemed to be the major thing that made the difference. In time, the terror settled down. My condition, which once again waxed and waned, gave me periods when I felt good, and periods when I didn't. Time eventually got me off Amantadine, and time slowly subdued Edmund. And after enough time, I embarked on my journey back to work. By Thanksgiving of 2020 things started to level out to a manageable place.

Before returning to work, I asked Dr. Kurtis, "What am I going to do moving forward?"

He looked at me and said, "You're going to wait and see."

Oh, God, I so don't want to hear that, I thought. I was so sick of that fucking word "wait." Why did I have to have a disorder that was wait and see? I never did well with wait and see. I hated to have to wait and see.

"I don't want to hear that," I blurted out.

"There's no other way," he responded.

COVID had shut down the drug program I was running, so I spent my days at my desk in the mental health unit with nothing much to do. To keep the facility open, the jail was running at the bare minimum and stopped all group and individual sessions.

My body still wasn't completely settled. I sat there and squirmed at my desk, trying to hide my movements from my colleagues. Luckily, some of the people I was working with were kind and understanding and took the brunt of the work that came in, leaving me plenty of time to scroll through my Facebook support groups and go for periodic walks around the jail to release my energy.

With nothing else to do, I decided to go through all my group material and get it organized for the big day when we would reopen the drug program. I was sitting in my cubicle and found a handout that I had given to many patients. It was a sheet on the concept of Radical Acceptance. I scrolled through it and reviewed the lines that I had read to others so many times before, but had never applied to myself. The sheet reminded me that life was worth living, even though bad things would happen. And it urged you to stop being angry at the fact that life was not what you anticipated.

As I read the words on that sheet about acceptance, they resonated differently with me that day. They hit at the core of what I was fighting. I felt my eyes tear up. Getting up from my desk, I walked into the bathroom to allow myself a moment to cry out my anger, but someone else was there. I settled for grabbing a paper towel to wipe my eyes and decided to go outside, telling my colleagues I was going for a cigarette.

As I left the jail, I went to my car, laid my head on the steering wheel, and let my angry tears flow. The handout's words kept ringing in my head, and I lost it that day. I had been avoiding this word for so long: *acceptance*. I didn't want to accept this. "Who the hell would want to accept this?" I shouted at the sky. *Why was acceptance the theme of this disorder? What about healing? Move past? Finished and over?*

That evening when I got home, I went for a walk. The word *acceptance* kept running through my brain. It was a cold afternoon with nothing but vultures flying in the sky. I like vultures. For most, they're a symbol of death. To me, death also means a cleansing, a chance for something new to form, and that's the symbolism I have always seen in those birds.

I started to think about all the time that had gone by and how much time Edmund had taken from me. I reflected on what I wanted my life to be and how this disorder had kept me trapped in my mind. I contemplated what it would look like if I were to accept this. Did I have a choice? Well, I did. I could kill myself, but is that what I wanted? And if I did accept my life as it was, did I want to spend it at the jail with other individuals whose lives had been taken away? What about my art? Theatre? Would those parts of my past never be again? Did I want this disorder to control every aspect of my life?

CHAPTER 34

"If You Get All These Problems . . ."

I want to pause my story for a moment to address some of the questions I often receive about my condition: "If you get all these problems when you go off the medication, why not just stay on the medication?" "Why did you taper your meds?" "Have you thought about just toughing it out and removing all the medications?" Another question I get: "When are you quitting smoking? Could that be contributing to this?" And my favorite: "Are you *sure* this isn't all in your head?" No matter how often I try to explain all of this to people, it never seems to click. But I'll try once again here.

Let's start with a basic concept. My brain receptors were damaged by the medications I was originally put on, and this damage is at a microscopic level that standard brain scans can't pick up. Technically, I'm brain damaged, but not in the traditional sense like a traumatic brain injury. The medicines I was placed on after the antipsychotics and the Reglan were meant to help manage the damage and give me a quality of life. At the time, this was the standard protocol. This is still the protocol for many. Edmund has now adapted to the combination of *all* the medications I'm taking. If this recipe is helping me, it would make sense to stay. This is not just about my pride or hope to get off medication, however.

These pills are complex and damage you in other ways. Benadryl is great when you have an occasional allergy or cold symptom. It's even good when you have an allergic reaction. In my case, Benadryl was originally added to counteract some of Edmund's wrath. When I took it every day, it started doing something different to my body.

In the past, when Scott rubbed my arm or ass, often he would say, "Wow, it feels like a baby's skin." I learned very early on to take care of my skin and moisturize daily. But all the moisturizing in the world couldn't undo the damage done by years of diphenhydramine drying out my skin. And new conditions appeared. Eczema and psoriasis came into my life and turned my once soft skin into a dry desert filled with cracking elbows and rashes. I know I can't completely blame it on the little pink pill. Smoking probably contributed just as much.

Smoking and nicotine are fun to think about when it comes to Edmund. In an effort to try and extend my life and start working on my singing voice again, I attempted to cut back and eliminate cigarettes. My once beautiful tenor sound had become that of a raspy baritone. When I tried to cut back about half of what I smoked per day, the simple removal of cigarettes caused the reoccurrence of intense akathisia and tics.

Dr. Lewis and Dr. Kurtis reminded me of my dopamine receptors, their role in movement, and how nicotine also affects dopamine. Dopamine doesn't just give you pleasurable feelings; it also affects your body's ability to regulate your movements. This is similar to Parkinson's patients, where a lack of dopamine is partially responsible for the movements you see in them. When people ask me about quitting, I have to remind them that the dopamine receptors in my brain are partially damaged, and quitting doesn't work so easily.

"What about patches, gum, vaping?" others will ask. They don't deliver nicotine the same way a cigarette does, and they don't seem to have the same effect on *my* dopamine system. Others, however, may have a different experience, but Edmund doesn't like these, and believe me, I've tried them all. I'm not making an excuse to not quit smoking, even though it probably sounds like that. If I currently want to quit, I have to cut back much slower, cigarette by cigarette, so as not to agitate Edmund.

As for Ativan, yes, at first it might calm you down, but there comes a point when your body gets used to it. Ativan hasn't helped my anxiety in years. I don't think it ever did. Some have argued that long-term benzodiazepine use can be associated with memory loss. I can certainly attest to this being true for me. My memory used to be great, but ever since this process started, my memory has turned to shit. I am constantly asking Scott, "What did we do last weekend? What was that restaurant we went to?"

I can forget just about anything if I'm not careful enough. Scott can always jolt my memory back into place, but I never know what I'm going to forget. If something or someone really didn't leave an impression on me, it will be forgotten.

Here's the other huge problem with benzodiazepines like Ativan: they are only supposed to be used for a short period of time—maybe two weeks. Long-term benzodiazepine use isn't generally the way to go. But what about people like myself who have been on them for years and are using them to help manage the symptoms of another condition caused by medications?

Long-term benzodiazepine use and discontinuing them requires a book all of its own, and I won't get into a long discussion about that here. I will say that it is a very difficult problem in the medical community. Many people are put on benzodiazepines and take them as prescribed, while others struggle with true addiction and have abused them. This further complicates the issue, because the latter has dominated the general population's and medical community's belief about benzodiazepines and the people who use them. Whenever I see a new doctor, there is an instantaneous assumption that I am a drug addict seeking pills. "You know I won't prescribe these pills for you?" they say.

Understandably, doctors want to get people off benzodiazepines, and, believe me when I say, most patients want off them as well. People will try to stop, but usually it's quite difficult, because their bodies and brains have become physically dependent on the drug to survive. For long-term benzo users, tapering the medication needs to happen over a long period of time and at a rate that is tolerable for the patient. Some people have been on them for so long that they may not be able to taper them in a traditional sense, if ever.

Not everybody gets taken off these pills with the optimal taper period for that patient. In accordance with traditional guidelines, well-intentioned doctors and detox facilities try to taper individuals who have been on benzodiazepines long-term in about six to eight weeks. Not-so-well-intentioned or informed doctors will remove the pills even faster. When this happens, it can cause some people to have a protracted withdrawal (a withdrawal that goes on much longer than anticipated), where individuals can have movement-related issues, like akathisia and other horrifying symptoms that can last for months and years, completely disabling them. Some people are never able to recover fully. There are numerous stories of people who have killed themselves because they were rapidly taken off a benzo.

So, what does this mean for people like me? Remember, the benzo-diazepine I am on is part of the combination helping to manage the original damage by the offending medication. Still, there is a good chance I could also be dependent on them. Do I stay on them or try to remove them? There's no clear consensus on this. Are they helping to regulate the damage done by the first pills, or am I dependent and unable to get off? Are both true? Is neither true? Does it even matter? You've seen what happens when I try to remove them: it paralyzes me—be it dependence or a reemergence from the original damage. What should I do?

A scenario of being rapidly tapered could be my fate as well if I don't have a doctor willing to work with me. In fact, now that I look back, the image of me being forced to taper probably played a part in my subconscious, which motivated my attempt to get off the benzodi-azepines in the first place. I have to recognize that Dr. Lewis won't be available to me forever. And, let's not forget that benzodiazepines are schedule IV narcotics. Laws and regulations are constantly changing on how these drugs are prescribed.

Then there is Trileptal, originally prescribed for a bipolar misdiagnosis and kept in Edmund's cocktail because it may have helped with my anxiety. It never appeared to cause problems . . . until it started causing problems. Trileptal messes with your electrolytes. I can't tell you how many times I've had low sodium at what could be considered dangerous levels because of that pill. Once, when I was hospitalized, they wouldn't release me until my sodium level rose. To try and raise my sodium, every morning I now drink a thirty-two-ounce bottle of electrolyte water to keep the fluids flowing through my system.-

As I rewrite this section in the final hour before releasing this book to the world, I just discovered that I have high blood pressure. My sodium is low, but my blood pressure is high. How the fuck does that work? I wish I could eat a bag of chips and call it a day, but it's not that simple. I've had to be referred to a nephrologist to make sure my kidneys aren't damaged from years of low sodium. The simplest of answers would be to remove some of the Trileptal. We have tried that, and Edmund was not happy with me.

It never ends, and it's not just the combination of medicines themselves. I have to be cautious about potential future medications, too. Remember the fungal infection that had invaded my ass more recently? It spread to my left armpit, and my dermatologist had to put me on a five-week regimen of Fluconazole. This is standard treatment for most people, but it affected my body's absorption of Ativan. The Ativan was going through my body faster than usual, which meant that I was going through an unintentional taper. To get the infection to clear, for several weeks I had to endure extra movements. Once again, I had to level out my brain.

When the COVID-19 vaccine was available and we were told that it would be mandatory in order to do certain things, I was filled with horror and panic at the thought of having to inject something into my body. *An untested vaccine going into my body and possibly setting Edmund off?*

There were no reports or data available on how this vaccine might affect a niche population like mine. Dr. Kurtis warned me that vaccines were known to trigger temporary movement disorders, because they can affect brain receptors. However, he encouraged me to get it. "Which outcome would be worse?" he said. That's a really hard question to answer with this disorder, and it was an incredibly difficult decision to make.

I'm not anti-vaccine. Before this, I would have gladly taken any vaccine. But now it would have to be weighed against the movement disorder and my current medicines. I eventually did get it—all of the doses. With each one, Edmund got set off, causing more movements. It actually got bad enough for me to briefly go back on the Amantadine.

As I said in the beginning, medication and I have a very complicated relationship. Anything that can affect my brain or nervous system must be thought about before it goes into my body. Do you know how many things can affect your nervous system and brain? The answer is everything, from stress and certain foods to caffeine to some types of exercise. Medicine? Very few of them don't affect the brain. Whatever the hell happened to my brain has made it nearly impossible for me to take even the most basic medications.

Other medicines I have taken that aren't traditionally associated with movement disorders have also brought about symptoms. Once, I tried taking a generic version of Vitamin C. That little pill brought back movements. I'm not saying Vitamin C causes movement disorders, but whatever damage was done to my brain has made it difficult for me to take even the simplest of pills. My body will often reject everything.

The big question: "Is this all in your head?" I still get this one. The subtext of what people are usually asking me when they say this is that the symptoms I'm experiencing are made up or that they're psychosomatic in nature. When I try to explain what's happening to me with a new doctor, I usually get the whole, "Oh wow, I've never heard of that," which is soon followed by an eye roll. I know what they're thinking:

"You're going to be one of *those* patients—the difficult ones who won't just take the pill and shut up. I deserve a Tony if I can make this all up, and I'd be happy to accept that award.

Psychosomatic—I have a hard time with that word, but I can see why people would think I have a somatic symptom disorder. Somatic disorders have symptoms that can't be explained medically, and patients often refuse to accept the facts in front of them. If you were to look at my story on the surface, I could see how it might appear that way. When I was first going through this ordeal, I had a hard time accepting what the doctors were telling me, and yes, I did see quite a few of them. But that was only because no doctor was listening to me, and they rejected everything I was trying to tell them. When Dr. Kurtis listened and explained my condition properly, while I was cautious about accepting his diagnosis due to a mistrust of doctors, I didn't dismiss his theory. What would my life have looked like if I had believed Dr. Baldisseri's or Dr. Pavlichuk's impression of me? I may never have left the psych ward.

Dr. Lewis and I have had very open and candid conversations about my mental health, and I have always trusted him to tell me the truth, even when I don't want to hear it. I have asked him about this somatic predicament. He never once doubted what he saw. Similar conversations have been had with Dr. Kurtis, and he concurred.

No, the research doesn't seem to support a somatic disorder. For a somatic disorder to be present, there can't be a better explanation for the symptoms. There is a better explanation. Hard data proves that akathisia and tardive dyskinesia can be permanent conditions caused by medications. It's right on the labels of the boxes of medications I took.

Still don't believe me? Go ahead and educate yourself by reading the now numerous amounts of legitimate, peer-reviewed research articles and teach yourself about D2, D3, D4 and GABA receptors in the brain, and all of these other types of neurological components. The articles are a lazy beach day type of read.

I think what people *really* have a difficult time understanding isn't so much that I have this disorder, but rather that my symptoms and reactions don't fit the textbook version of what is expected. But, in contrast, does every cancer patient have the same experience? Does every person who gets the flu need bed rest the same way? Does every medicine work for everyone equally?

I once had a gastrointestinal doctor say to me when questioning the validity of my tardive dyskinesia: "You're not moving *now*."

Seriously, I thought. *It doesn't work that way.* These gastrointestinal guys need to stop looking at assholes all day, lest they continue to become one themselves.

I don't want to give these nonbelievers any more attention in my life, and I've made a conscious effort to distance myself from them. I know they are misinformed and look at the world through a very narrow and controlled lens. So they can go ahead and call it somatic or whatever they want, but I'm going to call it: advocating for my health. And if I'm wrong and truly that insane and making this all up, then lock me up and throw away the key. Lord knows that would be a lot easier than having to listen to people's belittling comments.

This I will admit: Some of what could be going on may be a response to trauma. That is a possibility. My body might be responding physically in the present to my past, especially when it comes to trying a new pill. I wish people could spend thirty seconds in my mind and body when I have to take a new pill or try and remove one. Or when Edmund starts causing me agitation. I am always brought back to those early moments when this first occurred, and I feel like I am reliving this experience all over again.

Nevertheless, assuming you do believe me, here's the big dilemma I'm left to ponder regarding my condition. The medicines I'm currently on are partially causing it. This was truer with the antipsychotics. But if you remove the medicine, as I did, that causes it. And if you raise the dosage or add another medicine, that can cause it as well.

What does this current medication routine do for me? At this point, all these pills do is maintain equilibrium in my brain to give me some quality of life. I have two choices. One is to stay on the pills and "function," as it was so nicely put to me years ago. If I do that, I'll have to deal with the intermittent withdrawal from being on a benzodiazepine long-term. There will be days when the pills will make me more anxious, days when the pills won't seem to work. They will never fully keep the symptoms at bay, but the hope is that, with enough time, my body will continue to adjust. The pills will be an extension of me. This scenario is entirely dependent on Dr. Lewis or another doctor continuing to prescribe this current regimen and praying that I don't get rapidly tapered off some of these pills one day.

My other option is to continue to try and taper, as I've done before. But this time, do it slower than I ever have over the course of years, taking out fractions per year, if even that, with the hope that my brain will level out and adjust with each minuscule taper. Perhaps I do this by using a compounding pharmacy or another non-traditional method for removal. By doing this, the hope would be that, although we would upset Edmund somewhat, it would not be to the extent that he would disable me. The fear, however, is that if my body does not adjust, it would leave me in a place where I would be unable to do anything but tic and move incessantly, with the possibility of going in and out of periods of terror. There's also the danger of getting into a medical emergency like a car accident. The ER and hospital will give me my pills, but they won't be able to cut the pill to whatever dose I'm at. If I'm on .8752mg of Ativan, I will have to go up or down. Edmund probably won't like that either.

So the next time someone wants to ask me one of these questions, I'd like to ask them, "What would you do? Would any one of these options seem satisfactory to you? Would you stay on the pills or remove them? Would you ever take another pill again? Would you quit smoking? How would you feel about having to weigh this all out?" This is the reality I'm forced to ponder in my current life. And this was the reality I was being forced to accept back then.

CHAPTER 35
Goodbye

For a month after I found the Radical Acceptance sheet, I mulled over what to do going forward. Before making any decision, I planned and talked with Yulia and Scott, running and rerunning the numbers. Fear overcame me, and at one point I even tried to talk myself out of taking the leap and making changes. My former boss eased my worry when he said, "It's not like you're making a six-figure salary. If private practice doesn't work out for you, there will always be a ton of other jobs that will be willing to underpay and abuse you."

Finally, one morning I walked down the hall to my boss's office. She was typing away on her computer. I stood at the doorway and took one more deep breath before knocking.

"Can I talk to you?" I asked.

"Sure, come in," she said, smiling, having no clue of what I was about to do.

She saw the piece of paper that I held in my hand and said, "What is that?"

"I'm . . ."

". . . No!" she said. "We can tear that right up."

In April 2021, I gave my notice. It was time to work through my fear and pursue what I had originally set out to do when I entered the field of social work. My goal was to try and live as normal a life as possible and see my dream full circle: start my private practice; create art on my own terms; possibly return to acting—also on my own terms. Time, that awful word, was being wasted; I didn't want to waste any more and was determined to live my life as fully as I could.

Following my departure from my job, a day that I had thought about but tried not to fixate on, arrived. I learned that Dr. Kurtis was retiring. He was an older man, and I had anticipated that this would happen, but I had hoped it would be a lot further off in the distant future. I would have to accept that I would no longer receive his guidance. He made sure I was situated with a new specialist who understood my condition and spoke with them regarding current and future treatment. I wouldn't have let him leave if he hadn't.

The final day we met was incredibly difficult. I did my best to contain my emotions from taking over, putting on a fake smile, and congratulating him on his retirement. He told me how proud he was of me starting my private practice and said that I was an excellent social worker who would help lots of people. As I listened, the tears started to bubble up. I asked him about his next steps and what he was planning on doing in retirement, typical conversational banter. As our session came to an end, I couldn't help but ask him one last time: "Do you think I should ever try to taper again?"

Dr Kurtis replied in a reassuring tone. "The brain wants to heal itself. Don't forget that. The brain wants to heal. I don't know if you should try again, but I think your body and your brain will let you know."

Unable to hold back my feelings any longer, I broke down crying. Dr. Kurtis had been a pivotal part of this process, and I didn't want to lose him. I didn't want him to retire. When you find doctors you trust and who believe you, it's extremely hard to let them go. Finding him was a godsend. So many other individuals who struggle with this disorder have yet to find doctors who believe what they say they are experiencing. My thoughts went to Dr. Lewis, and I knew that one day I would be having this same conversation with him. My mind was all over the place.

Pulling myself together, I said, "Thank you for everything. You've helped me in so many ways."

It was unfortunate that this final session was virtual. Filled with so much gratitude for him and how he had been able to get me to this point, I would have wanted to give him a humongous hug. He shed a tear as he said, "You are going to get through this and live a normal life. Please remember that." As sad as I was to lose his guidance, I knew he was right. It would not be a normal life the way I used to define it; this would be a new version of normal. It was time for both of us to step into the next phases of our lives.

Unfinished, 20??, canvas, 10" x 10".

CHAPTER 36

Unfinished

The day had come when I would see my first patient as a full-time freelance practitioner. Excited and hopeful, I looked around at my basement, which had been turned into my office. I had done a lot to make this moment a reality. The trinkets I chose for my desk had meanings. My new computer was ready for teleconferencing. I thought how scary it all was, because it was so unknown, but here I was, doing it. Edmund was hanging around that day, but he had been caged in a box. He was trying to pop out but only managed to get a finger out that day.

For my whole life, I had let fear run the show. I feared my mother. I feared voicing my opinions to my partner. I feared what others thought. I feared quitting not just the jail, but also every job I ever had. I even feared my own brain. Fear had been running in the background of so many moments of my life, but as I sat in my office that first day, I realized that I was sitting amid fear and embracing it.

So often in my life, I attempted to combat fear by trying to control things over which I had no control. I tried to control my acting and art careers. I tried to control my anxiety by putting meds into my body and not stopping, even when a tiny voice inside of me said it was time to do so. I tried to control Edmund. During my movement disorder, I tried to control my paintbrushes, but I now realize how liberated my artwork would have been if I had loosened up my brush strokes. As I sat in my office that first day, about to see patients, there was a smile on my face because I was giving up control, choosing to give up control— not being forced to.

About to enter into a future that was anybody's guess, as I sat in my office giving up control, I did something I never thought I would allow myself to do: embrace uncertainty. I allowed myself to be in the midst of uncertainty and face the fear rather than run from it or try to control it—and I actually felt good doing that.

Dr. Kurtis' words to trust my body came to mind. The only way to handle uncertainty was to trust, to trust myself. That was so hard for me. My mother had taken away my ability to trust. The doctors who wouldn't listen to me, who didn't attempt to hear what I was saying, made trust in them nearly impossible. But then there were people like Scott, Nick, Dr. Zabel, Dr. Lewis, and Dr. Kurtis, who all showed me that trust and trusting myself was possible.

Looking back, Dr. Lewis was probably right. I do have some OCD. I don't have the classic rituals like washing my hands or counting, mine were more mental rituals: my need for constant reassurance, my need for absolute certainty, the endless questions that would invade my brain, questions that *had* to have answers. It made sense. With OCD, trust is a very hard thing. The irony is that my OCD may have partially brought Edmund into my life, yet in the moments when Edmund was trying to take over, my OCD and incessant need to know what was going on spurred me to research and find answers.

Quitting and letting go of the security of my job so I could have a full-time private practice wasn't just about making more money. It was about learning to trust in myself. I would never wish what I went through on myself or anyone else, but maybe this whole experience with the movement disorder needed to happen in order for me to reach this point.

Looking at my track record and where I've been, trying to trust isn't such a bad thing. I've done it before, and I often forget to consider my resilience. That was my father's gift and legacy to me, and Scott reinforced that. I got on stage, not just once, but multiple times in various cities. I put myself out there on the line. I moved across the country twice. I got through grad school. I'm working with Edmund. I didn't kill myself. I'm here to tell my story: I am fucking resilient. For me to have gone through all this and still be alive takes some fucking balls. For the time being, I get to sit in my office, a cup of decaf coffee in front of me, and I get to enjoy more and more moments of stillness.

I started painting again and have had my work accepted into art shows. Today it's less about being seen and making a living and more about what brought me to art in the first place. It's a chance to express myself and share my thoughts with the world. I really enjoy the stillness that enables me to do a painting and create the way I want again. For now, I can sit down and watch TV or sit with my patients and help them through their struggles. Even the stillness to write this piece feels great. I hope my body will allow me to be still enough to someday once again be on a stage. But for now, I take whatever stillness I get, and I never take it for granted.

I'd be lying if I said any of this was easy. Edmund doesn't make it easy. He lurks in the shadows, and he will make another big appearance one day. That I'm sure of. A big part of me also believes that Edmund may take my life someday, perhaps from cancer resulting from longtime smoking, being rapidly tapered off medication, or anything else he is capable of. What will Edmund look like as I continue to age? I try not to think about that or base my life on that, and I haven't lost hope that I will get my Shakespearian ending, where I get to say goodbye to Edmund and kill him—even if that's many years into the future. I do feel sorry for Edmund, both my Edmund and Shakespeare's. Neither asked to be born or to be illegitimate children. They were a product of their environment. But accountability is inevitable, and my Edmund will eventually have to pay for his wrongdoings. I hope it means he will be banished from my life forever.

I am practicing being okay with the thought that I might have to taper over a period of years, or even decades, or possibly never. A part of me still needs to believe that I can get off these pills, even if that may not be the reality. I need to believe that there will come a time when my body will let me know that I can try again—very, very slowly. Perhaps in the next decade new research will provide further options. I don't want to be a victim, and I do my best to push myself above and beyond the limits of this disorder. Sometimes I push too hard, and my body feels it, but other times, I am pleasantly surprised. For now, that's okay.

There is a final piece in this art series that has yet to be painted. I don't know what it is or what it will be. I know that I don't want to paint it until I've gotten more information from life. This blank canvas, like all blank canvases, is full of possibilities. And I'm truly trying to trust the process and enjoy the moments life is giving me, like sitting on my balcony and getting to watch the birds.

I love birds. We've always had a spiritual connection. They've come into my life at pivotal points, reminding me of the freedom of life. I enjoy being still and watching them in their wild madness as they fly around in our trees. I put a bird feeder outside my window and enjoy seeing all the different types that come to visit. My favorite is a woodpecker that I've named Fred. He finds the most ingenious ways to get the food from our squirrel-proof feeder, and he never gives up. These past couple of years robins have come to nest on our property. Now, I just let them be.

Epilogue

Medication-induced movement disorders are still misunderstood. We don't know enough about them. Why do they happen to some and not to others? Is there a genetic component? Is the terror that I and others have felt part of the condition, or does it deserve a category all its own? Way more research needs to be done. All we have to date is that it is "difficult to treat," and often misdiagnosed. I wish we could simply categorize all Side Effect Related Disorders as "SERD" and leave the details and semantics for individual cases. People experience all sorts of things when medications don't work the way they're supposed to. Maybe future generations of doctors will specialize in SERDs.

For now, prevention, to the extent that is possible, is the best answer. Further research and education will provide new answers. I never thought when this first happened to me that there would be a day I would see TV commercials for medications used to treat tardive dyskinesia. People who've seen these ads often ask, "Isn't that what you have?" Every person who asks gives me an opportunity to educate them about what's going on and explain the world of medication-induced disorders.

If there's only one thing you take away from this book, let it be this: Akathisia, tardive dyskinesia, dystonic reactions, medication-induced Tourette's, the overarching blanket term of tardive syndrome, and the more general medication-induced movement disorders are not made up. They're officially recognized. There's a whole section in the *Diagnostic and Statistical Manual of Mental Disorders (DSM)*.

Unfortunately, many doctors are not trained to look for medication-induced movement disorders. Some who do recognize them choose to ignore patients who don't fit into a classic textbook definition of what the disorders should look like. My heart goes out to the thousands of other niche communities of people who are struggling for answers to what is ailing them and who must plow through a multitude of doctors who want to label them as "crazy" because they don't fit into the typical medical model. One of the scariest things that can happen to a person when they recognize that something is not right with them is to be told, "You're lying" or, "You're anxious." It should not be the patient's responsibility to figure out their diagnosis. All too often patients must become the doctor and researcher to help make sense of what is happening inside of them. When patients are forced to take on these roles, it leads to needless, uninformed, and sometimes harmful experimentation that a person must undertake alone, without anyone to guide their care.

If you are part of the medical community and have stumbled upon this book, rather than dismissing or disbelieving what the patient is describing, I urge you to take the time to educate yourself about medication-induced movement disorders. Many health providers, including medical doctors, social workers, psychologists, counselors, and nurses, are not familiar with these disorders, yet this is not a new phenomenon. The research goes back to the development and introduction of psychiatric medications. You may be the patient's only hope to recognize what is going on in their body and help them deal with it.

Someone once asked me: "Do you think if you had better doctors this still would have happened to you?"

"Maybe," I responded. "But I'd also like to think that someone would have been able to catch this sooner, before it completely overtook my life."

When I was working at the jail, several inmates were experiencing medication-induced movement disorders, and I was able to recognize the signs when others didn't. They were lucky, and, armed with this new information, they consulted with their doctors and were able to get off the meds without any long-term damage. I can't tell you how many people have thanked me profusely after I suggested they stop taking medication because those medications were not what they needed. If you're a provider not familiar with how to recognize these disorders, tons of resources are available: online videos of patients, journal articles, and even a continuing education class now offered through MISSED (see Resources). I implore you to become a leader in this field.

If you are struggling with akathisia, tics, agitation, or combinations of them, know that you will get through the worst of it. I don't know how long it will take, but you will. If you're one of the lucky ones who have gotten off pills, I'm so happy for you. You will be able to put your Edmund to bed and move beyond his torture.

For the rest of you, I share my experience in the hope that it will help in some way. Everyone's journey through these disorders will be different, but I can tell you that the people I've seen who get better are the ones who wait and let time do its thing.

Sometimes people must stay on medication far longer than they would like. Some can taper quickly, others, not so much. That's a hard thing to hear when you're being tortured. Some people will want to try other pills to help alleviate symptoms, and they will work. Others will try the same pill and won't have any relief. Many won't ever touch a pill again. There is no one way to manage the symptoms of these disorders. Everyone will have to find their own unique path. When you do find that path, own it, embrace it, and don't go down it alone.

My blood curdles when I see advertisements on TV for antipsychotics being marketed to the general public and I hear the voiceover say in happy and calm tones: "May cause uncontrollable muscle movements, which may become permanent." But profits drive the pharmaceutical industry, and that is not necessarily in the best interest of the public. It would be easy and naïve of me to say to everyone, "Don't take these pills," but, as a talk therapist, I know that the same pills that took so much away from my life and that of others have given life back to somebody else.

As much as I want to be angry with every doctor who prescribes these pills and the drug companies that make them, all that would do is keep me trapped in a vicious cycle of resentment and bitterness, destroying my life in other ways. These pills do work for many. And there are times in our lives when we are going to need pills. There's no way around it. Pills, however, should be a last resort and taken and prescribed with extreme caution. Often that is not the case when it comes to mental health meds. We need to stop overmedicating people.

Needless to say, if these pills worked so well, I would be out of business as a therapist; and on the flip side, if these pills worked so well, people would be more compliant and stay on them. While working in corrections, I often saw repeat offenders come in and out of jail mainly because they stopped taking their medication. One of the biggest reasons people don't want to stay on mental health meds: side effects. The meds may be the best option we have right now, but surely we can shoot for better as the decades go on. The formulas for mental health medications haven't changed much. They're the same types of drugs with different names or branding makeovers.

If you're considering taking a pill to *manage* your mental health, before you go that route, you might want to try talk therapy first. But, if you want to get the most out of that experience, you must be willing to put in the work. It can feel incredibly daunting and overwhelming to work on yourself, especially when you're not feeling your best. It's hard, but you cannot avoid the necessary work required, and it can be worth it. Reminder: the key word here is *manage* your mental health, not eliminate symptoms or feelings.

Oftentimes when a person first sees a mental health professional their goal is to get rid of a feeling. But feelings are just your body's way of giving you information. It can be incredibly difficult to learn how to manage negative feelings, because many people are not taught exactly how to deal with feelings growing up. Identifying and managing your feelings will be the most difficult task you can undertake, but the rewards are more beneficial than any pill will ever give you, and you will feel more empowered and resilient for going through the process.

If you're struggling with your mental health and must take medication, start slowly. These are very complex pills, and we're still not sure how all of them work in the bodies and brains of different people. And this isn't just limited to psychiatric medications. Certain decongestants and plenty of other medications have been linked to cases of medication-induced movement disorders.

Find a doctor you trust, especially if you're going to take medication. Most in-network doctors are overworked, overbooked, and have long wait times to see them. There's a good chance you will get lost inside that spectrum. Self-pay physicians and psychiatrists don't usually have as many patients, but even some of them can be second-rate and expensive. Don't even get me started on the cost of healthcare in the U.S.! The important thing is that you get someone who will listen to you and your concerns. Don't be afraid to ask questions, like "How do you handle adverse reactions to medications?" and "What's your emergency policy?" If it's not a right fit, get the fuck out of there.

A great doctor is one who is willing to look between the lines. One who can admit when they don't know and will help you find the solutions or point you to people who might. Find one who knows how to listen. And if you are a doctor, who perhaps did not listen and hear what a patient in distress was describing, I hope you will hear this as a wake-up call to reorient your thinking. Dr. Lewis has admitted to me that we got lucky, that he didn't know all the answers and still doesn't know all the answers. Dr. Kurtis said similar things over the years. I knew that they didn't have all the answers or keys to my health, but it was their ability to *listen* that made them such great doctors. Listening requires responsive communication that leads to understanding and empathy. Maybe we should all learn to listen better.

During the second round with this disorder, I was watching one of my mentors speak on Facebook for a Benzo Awareness Day Live Stream event. He, too, was afflicted with a movement disorder. He said something so incredibly powerful that I want to quote him to sum up my journey: "I will never be grateful for this, but I will learn from it and take away its lessons." . . . Ditto.

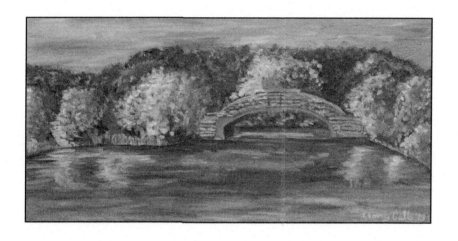

Verona Park, 2023, oil on canvas, 12" x 36".

Acknowledgments

This book would not have been possible without the help of the following individuals. For all of you, I am eternally grateful.

To my editors, Louise D. Stahl and Don Weise: Thank you for your exceptional work in helping me see my vision come to life. And a special thank you to the amazingly talented Sondra Beaulieu, my Editor in Chief. I would not have done this book without your eyes to guide me through this process. You are the best and your tireless efforts have not gone unnoticed. Thanks for not editing *me* out of my book.

To my book and cover designer Glen Edelstein—your efforts in bringing this project together worked beautifully. Thanks for all your hard work and patience with me.

Marc Cashman—Thank you for your wonderful audio narration in the audio production of the book. And thank you, KC Styles, for your music in the book.

Also, a special thanks to Gregory G. Allen and Lisa Ahfeld, whose invaluable input has helped me in more ways than you will ever know.

Dr. Lewis and Dr. Kurtis: I wouldn't be where I am today if it wasn't for your support and guidance. I am eternally grateful to you both.

Nick and Yuliya: Your wisdom, guidance, and patience throughout the years have always been a rock for me. Thank you. I don't know what I would do without the two of you.

And to my father: Dad, you will always be the strongest person I know. Your support has always been at the foundation of everything I do.

And finally, to my partner in life, Scott: I will never be able to express in words how much your love, support, and patience have meant to me throughout all of our years together. I love you always.

Resources

The Akathisia Alliance for Education and Research
https://akathisiaalliance.org

MISSD (The Medication-Induced Suicide Prevention and Education Foundation)
https://missd.co
P.O. Box 10107
Chicago, IL 60610

The Benzodiazepine Information Coalition
https://www.benzoinfo.com
P.O. Box 1433
Venice, FL 34284

Mad in America
https://www.madinamerica.com
763 Massachusetts Ave.
Suite 3
Cambridge, MA 02139

The Dystonia Medical Research Foundation
https://dystonia-foundation.org
1 E. Wacker Drive
Suite 1730
Chicago, IL 60601

The Tourette Association of America
https://tourette.org
42-40 Bell Blvd.
Suite #507
Bayside, NY 11361

The National Organization for Rare Disorders
https://rarediseases.org
1900 Crown Colony Drive
Suite 310
Quincy, MA 02169

About the Author

Lenny Gallo is a writer, artist, and clinical social worker. His artwork has been featured in galleries worldwide, and his essays and articles have been featured in professional journals and trade papers. In addition to his art and writing, Lenny works as a therapist, specializing in the treatment of OCD, trauma, and anxiety disorders. Originally from Chicago, he now resides in New Jersey.

Printed in Great Britain
by Amazon

56359233R00158